See What Others Have Said About *Treatment Alternatives for Children*

"More and more parents are looking to integrate conventional and natural treatments for their kids. Dr. Rosen and Jeff Cohen provide a comprehensive book that doctors and parents can rely on for science-based treatment alternatives. I incorporate natural remedies into my pediatric practice whenever possible and will keep this book handy to help guide my decisions."
—Dr. Bob Sears, Pediatrician and author of *The Portable Pediatrician*

"Pediatrics is about treating the whole child, not just 'an ear' or 'a cold.' I often find that the conventional medicine I've been taught doesn't give me the tools I need to offer to parents to prevent and treat their kids. Dr. Rosen and Jeff Cohen offer a truly integrative approach of treatment alternatives to treat children of all ages."
—Jay N. Gordon, MD, FAAP, Assistant Professor of Pediatrics, UCLA Medical School

"Dr. Larry Rosen is the real deal! He lives and breathes the holistic lifestyle he recommends to families. He is widely recognized as one of the foremost authorities on the safe and evidence-based integration of complementary therapies into pediatric care and also well known for his commitment to leading the way in the "greening" of healthcare. In teaming up with Jeff Cohen, successful author and holistic parent, together they've written an invaluable resource for parents and healthcare professionals alike."
—Timothy Culbert, MD, FAAP, Medical Director: Pediatric Integrative Medicine, Ridgeview/Two Twelve Medical Center

"Dr. Rosen is the best pediatrician I've ever come across. Not only is he knowledgeable and kind but he really does look at your child from all angles and comes up with the most effective holistic remedies and treatments."
—Aidan Quinn, actor and parent

"Parents are increasingly turning to natural, non-toxic remedies for themselves and their families but are often uncertain where to start. This handy, practical guide by Dr. Rosen and Jeff Cohen helps parents to navigate their way into natural healing safely and effectively. It is a must-have for holistic-minded parents and for all parents who want to be informed about the healing options available for common childhood ailments."
—Nancy Massotto, Founder & Executive Director, Holistic Moms Network, www.holisticmoms.org

"Dr. Rosen is a national leader in integrative care for children. His work, with co-author Jeff Cohen, is thoughtful, based on sound scientific evidence, and ultimately on deep care and respect for children and families. I plan to use this book extensively in my practice and teaching."
—Kathi J Kemper, MD, MPH, author of *The Holistic Pediatrician, Mental Health Naturally,* and *Addressing ADD Naturally*; Director, Center for Integrative Medicine, Wake Forest School of Medicine

"This is a must-have resource for parents who want the best for their children's health. *Treatment Alternatives for Children* covers everything from colic to bruises and does the work for you by giving the conventional remedy and treatment alternative in chart form. Who can argue with olive oil and chamomile as a first line of defense for your little one? Stick with nature, it always knows best."
—Stacey Antine, MS, RD, founder of HealthBarn USA

"Dr. Rosen has the unique ability to inform, educate and re-assure in the language that parents speak. *Treatment Alternatives for Children* is an indispensable resource for Moms and Dads who are enlightened—and those who want to be."
—Bob Klapisch, Columnist (*Bergen Record*), Author, TV Analyst

"What a tremendous gift for parents and children! By comparing conventional to alternative treatments side-by-side, Rosen and Cohen give families what they need to make informed choices about common ailments to fit their particular situation and approach to health. *Treatment Alternatives* is practical, balanced, and full of health. A treasure!"
—Alan Greene, MD, FAAP, author of *Raising Baby Green*; Founding President, Society for Participatory Medicine

Treatment Alternatives *for* Children

Lawrence Rosen, MD, and Jeff Cohen

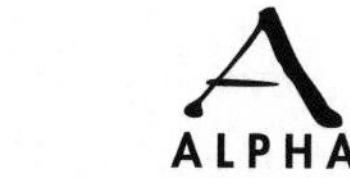

ALPHA
A member of Penguin Group (USA) Inc.

For Laura, the love of my life. —Dr. Rosen

For my loving parents Janis and Bert Cohen, as well as Carol, Gabriel, and Sienna, my amazing wife and kids I will love forever and a day. —Jeff Cohen

ALPHA BOOKS

Published by Penguin Group (USA) Inc.

Penguin Group (USA) Inc., 375 Hudson Street, New York, New York 10014, USA • Penguin Group (Canada), 90 Eglinton Avenue East, Suite 700, Toronto, Ontario M4P 2Y3, Canada (a division of Pearson Penguin Canada Inc.) • Penguin Books Ltd., 80 Strand, London WC2R 0RL, England • Penguin Ireland, 25 St. Stephen's Green, Dublin 2, Ireland (a division of Penguin Books Ltd.) • Penguin Group (Australia), 250 Camberwell Road, Camberwell, Victoria 3124, Australia (a division of Pearson Australia Group Pty. Ltd.) • Penguin Books India Pvt. Ltd., 11 Community Centre, Panchsheel Park, New Delhi—110 017, India • Penguin Group (NZ), 67 Apollo Drive, Rosedale, North Shore, Auckland 1311, New Zealand (a division of Pearson New Zealand Ltd.) • Penguin Books (South Africa) (Pty.) Ltd., 24 Sturdee Avenue, Rosebank, Johannesburg 2196, South Africa • Penguin Books Ltd., Registered Offices: 80 Strand, London WC2R 0RL, England

International Standard Book Number: 978-1-61564-181-9
Library of Congress Catalog Card Number: 2012930860

14 13 12 8 7 6 5 4 3 2 1

Interpretation of the printing code: The rightmost number of the first series of numbers is the year of the book's printing; the rightmost number of the second series of numbers is the number of the book's printing. For example, a printing code of 12-1 shows that the first printing occurred in 2012.

Printed in the United States of America

Publisher: Marie Butler-Knight
Associate Publisher/Acquiring Editor: Mike Sanders
Executive Managing Editor: Billy Fields
Development Editor: Mark Reddin
Senior Production Editor: Janette Lynn
Copy Editor: Jaime Julian Wagner
Cover & Book Designer: Rebecca Harmon
Layout: Brian Massey
Proofreader: John Etchison

ALWAYS LEARNING PEARSON

Contents

Alphabetical List of Ailments

Foreword

Nothing is more important than our health—except the health of our children. From the time they are infants and through young adulthood, nearly everything our sons and daughters eat, drink, inhale, swallow, or rub on their skin is determined by their parents, often at the advice of a pediatrician. Over the last decade, as the founder and president of the Deirdre Imus Environmental Health Center, I have worked to help raise awareness of the dangers posed by toxins in cleaning agents, food, personal care products, medications, vaccinations, and much more. I can count on one hand the number of people I've met who are as passionate as I am about the health of our children, and ensuring their physical, mental, and emotional health is a priority. Dr. Lawrence Rosen is one of those people.

Dr. Rosen's dedication to integrative medicine—to treating *The Whole Child*, as the name of his pediatric practice implies, and not just the part that hurts—is evident in every page of *Treatment Alternatives for Children.* Dr. Rosen and Jeff Cohen, a writer and holistic-minded father in his practice, present integrative views of both doctor and parent throughout the book, a nod to the healing power of the doctor-family relationship. I met Dr. Rosen more than five years ago, when we found ourselves on the same side of many children's health issues. Immediately, I knew I had met a kindred spirit. Information is key to the way Dr. Rosen practices medicine, and this book is chock-full of it. Because approaching medicine from a holistic—rather than reactive—standpoint requires a deep understanding of the way all the various systems and parts of the body work in tandem to create or negate health.

As a pediatrician, Dr. Rosen, who is also the medical adviser to the Deirdre Imus Environmental Health Center, is on the front lines of the epidemics threatening our kids: autism; allergies; asthma: ADD; ADHD; obesity; diabetes; premature births; and many other chronic illnesses. He also understands the impact various environmental factors—everything from air pollution to contaminated personal care products—can have on a child's health. Rather than immediately prescribe a potentially harmful drug for an ailing child, Dr. Rosen seriously considers each unique situation and considers the most practical solution.

In this book, you'll find a comprehensive guide to treating common ailments in your infant, toddler, child, or teen using natural methods, like oils and herbs and supplements. There are lists of salves for problems at each age, along with detailed lists of likely and unlikely allergic reactions to remedies both conventional and homeopathic. You'll even hear directly from parents like Jeff about specific remedies that have helped their own kids. *Treatment Alternatives for Children* is really all you could ever want or need in an alternative treatments guide.

And, as many people have discovered firsthand, Dr. Rosen, whom I like to call a "Green Doctor," is really all a parent or patient could ever want in a pediatrician. I can understand why Jeff, his holistic co-author, was drawn to Dr. Rosen's "green pediatrics" approach. He makes everyone feel comfortable from the second they walk through the door of The Whole Child Center. His personality perfectly suits his pediatric patients: by speaking directly *to them* (and not to their looming parents), Dr. Rosen gets to know his charges and, in that way, takes their wellness personally.

Because what is practicing medicine about, if not wellness? As you will see in this book, the remedies Dr. Rosen and Jeff Cohen recommend are not merely curative—they are preventive, often enhancing a child's overall health. While many of his colleagues concentrate on treating illness and managing disease, Dr. Rosen focuses on the entirety of his patient. It's unclear to me when we stopped demanding this sort of attention from our doctors, but if Dr. Rosen is any indication of things to come, then I am nothing short of thrilled for the future of medicine in this country—for us, for our kids, for our health.

Deirdre Imus,
President and Founder of The Deirdre Imus Environmental Health Center™ at Hackensack University Medical Center and Co-Founder/ Director of the Imus Cattle Ranch for Kids with Cancer.

Introduction

It's 6:52 A.M. on a Tuesday and my four-year-old son awakes with puffy eyes. He looks like a knocked-out boxer in the post-fight press conference.

"Daddy, if I'm awake, why can't I see anything?" You've got to love toddler questions.

"Well, Gabe, I'm guessing you have pinkeye." Anyone with young kids knows it's never one-and-done with questions.

"Did I play with anything pink yesterday? Aren't my eyes brown?" Could I get orange eye 'cause that's my favorite color?"

Flash ahead two hours and we leave the eye doctor with prescription in hand. The diagnosis is not pinkeye, it's pollen allergies. The scribbled blue paper calls for ocular steroid eye drops.

Flash ahead another hour and I'm dangling the first drop over a frightened, wincing little boy. Landing the first drop will be harder than typing on a BlackBerry with your knuckles. First drop lands on his shirt. Second drop douses his forehead. Third drop cures the carpet but not my kid.

"Let's take a break before we finish the bottle." Perusing the label, I can't help but notice the warnings.

Warning #1: May cause elevated pressure inside the eye that can lead to vision damage.

Warning #2: May increase the risk of cataracts clouding the lens of the eye that can impair vision.

Whoa! I'm trying to cure the kid, not blind him! Does a 4-year-old need steroids? Didn't all those ballplayers experience back acne, bulging necks, hair loss, and anger management problems?

Maybe missing Gabe's eye was a blessing. I call Dr. Rosen, our holistic-minded pediatrician. "Try Optique, a homeopathic treatment for eye irritation. Let him lie down with his eyes closed, aim the drop at the inner corner of the eye, and ask him to blink a couple of times." No vision damage, no cloudy lens, no wrestling matches—count me in!

Gabe and I improve our eye drop accuracy and two days later he can see perfectly again. Welcome to the beginning of our journey from conventional to holistic parenting. Never again would my wife and I blindly fill prescriptions.

Weeks later I ran into our eye doctor at the grocery store and asked him about Optique. "Never heard of it," he responded. "It's a homeopathic alternative to steroid drops," I explained. Who knew eye doctors could have such blank stares!

An Integrative Approach

The puffy eye experience changed the way my wife and I looked at doctors. We realized conventional doctors know conventional treatments but holistic parents like ourselves want the total picture. Sadly, you can't find a holistic eye doctor, physical therapist, and gastroenterologist in every city.

Now I'm not here to tell you to ultimately pick the conventional or holistic choice. That's your job as a loving parent. I just want you armed with credible information when you need it—mainly, the point at which a doctor hands you the prescription. We're all busy. We all scan the internet for health information when we need it. But who wrote these articles? Is it an established medical professional or a bored, opportunistic teenager?

Meet Dr. Rosen

I've partnered with Dr. Lawrence Rosen, a renowned and board-certified pediatrician committed to family-centered, holistic childcare. He's a nationally recognized expert in Pediatric Integrative Medicine and understands the full spectrum of conventional and natural treatment options. That's the beauty of integrative medicine—it's not either/or but the best of both. Check him and his pediatric practice out at www.wholechildcenter.org and you'll understand why he's the right co-author for this book.

His practice is built around the Consortium of Academic Health Centers for Integrative Medicine's definition of integrative healthcare. "Integrative medicine is the practice of medicine that reaffirms the importance of the relationship between practitioner and patient; focuses on the whole person; is informed by evidence; and makes use of all the appropriate therapeutic approaches, healthcare professionals, and disciplines to achieve optimal health and healing." Not a bad philosophy for raising happy, healthy kids!

In fact, let's take a closer look at the key words that make up the definition of integrative pediatrics:

- **Relationship:** The bond and communication between pediatrician, child, and family is crucial both diagnostically and therapeutically.
- **Whole:** The mind, body, and spirit of the child are linked and need to be in balance for optimal health.
- **Evidence:** Integrative pediatricians are guided by their intuition and experience as well as research findings. They value individuality and understand that one size does not fit all.
- **Appropriate:** Risks considered safe for adults might not be safe for children. Integrative pediatricians value gentle, natural remedies whenever possible.
- **Optimal Health:** Integrative pediatricians focus on wellness and prevention with a strong belief in the innate healing capacity of children. Health is considered not just the absence of disease but also the presence of optimal functioning.

Talk about an all-encompassing approach to childcare! Bottom line: this book is not about conventional versus alternative treatments for kids. It's really integrative, discussing the pros and cons of both.

Medical and Parental Perspectives

Dr. Rosen as co-author lets you know a renowned pediatrician is fully behind the medical advice in this book. However, together we wanted to go one step beyond just medical opinions. We know parents often rely on other parents when seeking treatment recommendations.

So throughout this book we'll share the pediatric and parental perspective (both of us are loving and doting dads) on conventional versus natural treatments for kids. As the provider and receiver of treatment, we've got both viewpoints covered for you. We don't stop there! We've also enlisted advice from parents around the world on remedies they've successfully used for their kids. You'll see this in the "Parental Guidance" sidebars throughout the book.

How to Use This Book

Have you ever used an English-to-Spanish dictionary? You look up the word *table* and quickly discover it's *mesa* in Spanish. Well, think of this book as your conventional-to-natural dictionary. Here you'll find that a conventional treatment for allergies, like Benadryl, translates into a natural alternative called Sabadil.

We know you're super-busy running a household. We don't expect you to block off 72 hours and read this book cover to cover while sipping a latte and getting a foot rub from your spouse. Then again, you're probably due for a foot rub—so squeeze that in if you can.

We want to give you the exact information you need when you need it—mainly at the very point of making a medical decision for your child. So stuff this book in your diaper bag or glove compartment. Pull it out when you've got a conventional prescription in hand or a sick kid at home and want the natural alternative. You'll quickly see:

- The causes and symptoms of nearly 100 childhood ailments
- The conventional course of treatment for each ailment, including recommended dosage, active ingredients, and possible side effects

- A natural, homeopathic, and/or holistic alternative to the conventional treatment
- Two or three additional natural treatments to consider beyond the one highlighted for each ailment in the section called "Natural Selection"

For every ailment covered in this book you'll see a table with both the associated conventional remedy and treatment alternative. You can expect to see dosage information, how it works, potential side effects, and active ingredients. As a reminder, active ingredients are the ones responsible for the given effect advertised by the medication (i.e., to reduce coughing symptoms). Active ingredients are the part of the medication that does what the product is designed to do. Inactive ingredients (which are not listed in this book's tables) are used to create the medication's formulation (i.e., into a liquid, capsule, or pill). The actual amount of active ingredient in a given medication is often so small that inactive ingredients are needed to bulk up the product into an easy-to-use form for the patient.

While we did not have enough room in the tables to list inactive ingredients, as the parent you should be sure to review them before choosing a product for your child. Potentially harmful dyes and chemicals can be common inactive ingredients, so you'll want to check labels and ingredients to fully understand what your child is ingesting.

Ultimately, it's your kid—who are we to make a medical decision for you? If this book has done its job, you'll be armed with integrative choices to make your own informed medical decisions the next time your kid coughs, sneezes, aches, drips, limps, whimpers, itches, or cries.

What Ails Your Kid?

With nearly 100 ailments covered in this book, it can be daunting to find the right section for your child's condition. That's why we've created a twofold table of contents. First, the ailments are broken into categories, primarily by body parts and related conditions. That's why diaper rash and teething are in Chapter 1 on Baby Matters while acne and head lice are in Chapter 9 on Dermatological Dilemmas. Second, immediately after the categories, you'll find an alphabetical listing of every ailment and the associated page number.

In the Spotlight

At the end of each chapter you'll see one additional topic covered in the "Spotlight On" section. Look for photos throughout this book highlighting these spotlighted treatments and preventative measures. The purpose here is to emphasize an integrative topic that applies to the entire chapter. For example, look for probiotics in Chapter 2 on mouth-related ailments. And be sure to check out the spotlight on mind-body medicine in Chapter 6 on tummy troubles.

Celebrity Sound Off

Each chapter also kicks off with an original quote from holistic-minded celebrities and health experts. We reached out to them directly to better understand how they apply integrative medicine in their own lives (and the lives of their kids). Within chapters, we've also included professional pointers from nationally known integrative experts.

Sidebars Explained

Your ailment journey also includes multiple sidebars providing additional tips and new ideas to help you as parents make better-informed decisions. The three sidebar types you'll see throughout this book are:

Parental Guidance

Actual quotes from parents who have effectively used various treatment alternatives to improve their child's condition.

✓ Good to Know

Fun facts and statistics related to the conditions covered throughout the book that add scope and quantifiable data to the information presented.

Science Says

The scientific rationale explained by Dr. Rosen for each of the treatment alternatives covered in the book adds credibility to the recommendations.

At this point you understand the definition of integrative medicine. You've met Dr. Rosen. You know how to read and best use the book in front of you. All that's left is to answer one simple question. What ails you—or, more precisely, what ails your child?

Acknowledgments

Dr. Rosen: I always suspected I had a book in me, but it wasn't until Jeff Cohen approached me with a "couldn't-pass-it-up" offer that this dream became reality. Jeff deserves all the credit in the world for shepherding this labor of love to delivery. He and Carol are wonderful parents, and I thank them for partnering with me not only for their children's care but also for helping other parents through this book.

I owe much gratitude to the many practitioners who have offered nuggets of wisdom throughout the text to complement our work. Of equal value are the personal stories of parents; I thank them for sharing their own favorite remedies. The greatest lessons I have learned are courtesy of the children and families I have had the pleasure of serving. These families are daily inspiration for me and for my colleagues at The Whole Child Center. Nurse Karen and my pediatric associates are invaluable as we work together to keep kids healthy.

Finally, thank you to my family for their unwavering support. My parents, Barbara and Martin Rosen, have nurtured and inspired me more than any son could wish. My children, Matthew and Talia, provide me with daily reminders of why being a parent is one of the greatest joys in life. And to my wife, Laura, thank you simply for being you—the best partner in the whole wide world.

Jeff Cohen: Dr. Rosen really does treat the "whole child" and never makes you feel another patient is waiting. This book is a testament to Dr. Rosen's integrative approach to medicine. My children are healthier and happier thanks to him. He's a man of integrity, patience, and thoughtfulness. I'm proud to call him a co-author and friend.

Thank you to my wife and muse Carol. You always see my potential and never give up until I reach it. Thank you to my kids, Gabriel and Sienna, who offer unconditional love, hugs, and smiles. Thanks to my parents, Janis and Bert Cohen, for helping me through my own "growing pains" and making me the man I am today. It wasn't until I had my own kids that I finally realized and truly appreciated what it takes to raise a family. Thank you to my older sister Alyssa for breaking in our parents and easing those same growing pains. Thank you to my newer sister Diana for scrumptious short ribs and banana bread which fueled my late night writing. Thank you to Alice "Gram-Gram" Winitt who read one of my adolescent summer camp letters and predicted I'd someday be a published author.

Thank you to the Horvath and deBoer families for producing lifetime playmates in Samantha, Rebecca, Ari, and Julia. Thanks to Miriam for delicious cooking and unwavering loyalty. Thanks to Daniel for constant laughs and for loving Miriam. Thank you to Victor who despite no longer being here continues to show me how to turn obstacles into stepping stones.

Dr. Rosen and Jeff Cohen: Thank you to our super agents, Janet Rosen and Sheree Bykofsky, for championing this book from conception to the book shelf. You believed in this idea from day one and your passion brought this book to life. Thanks also to Mike Sanders, Mark Reddin, Janette Lynn, and the amazing team at Alpha Books/Penguin Group for guiding this book to market. Thank you to our technical editor Tamra Holtzer, although technically she is also a dear friend. Thanks to Jennifer Johnson, our researcher extraordinaire, for methodically looking up every dosage, side effect, and symptom in this book. Finally, thanks to Aimee Gatti for all the front-end book proposal research and inspirational motherly advice along the way.

Medical Disclaimer

INFORMATION CONTAINED IN THIS BOOK IS INTENDED AS AN EDUCATIONAL AID ONLY. INFORMATION IS NOT INTENDED AS MEDICAL ADVICE FOR INDIVIDUAL CONDITIONS OR TREATMENT AND IS NOT A SUBSTITUTE FOR A MEDICAL EXAMINATION, NOR DOES IT REPLACE THE NEED FOR SERVICES PROVIDED BY MEDICAL PROFESSIONALS OR INDEPENDENT DETERMINATIONS. INDIVIDUAL DOCTORS MUST MAKE THEIR OWN INDEPENDENT DETERMINATIONS BEFORE AUTHORIZING A COURSE OF ANY TREATMENT OR PRESCRIPTION. A PERSON'S INDIVIDUAL DOCTOR MUST DETERMINE WHAT IS SAFE AND EFFECTIVE FOR EACH INDIVIDUAL PERSON OR PATIENT. THE AUTHORS DO NOT ASSUME ANY RESPONSIBILITY OR RISK FOR THE USE OF ANY INFORMATION CONTAINED WITHIN THE BOOK. WHILE THE AUTHORS HAVE DONE THEIR BEST TO ENSURE FULL INTEGRITY THROUGHOUT ALL MEDIAS, THEY MAKE NO GUARANTEES WHATSOEVER REGARDING THE ACCURACY, COMPREHENSIVENESS, AND UTILITY OF THE WORK. THE AUTHORS PROVIDE NO ENDORSEMENT OF AND ARE NOT RESPONSIBLE FOR THE ACCURACY OR RELIABILITY OF ANY OPINION, ADVICE, OR STATEMENT MADE WITHIN THE BOOK OTHER THAN AUTHORIZED BY THE AUTHORS DIRECTLY. THE AUTHORS ARE NOT LIABLE FOR ANY LOSS OR DAMAGE CAUSED BY THE READER'S RELIANCE ON THE INFORMATION

Trademarks

1

Baby Matters

"More and more parents are turning to natural, holistic, and alternative approaches to health care. As this demand increases, more and more classically trained physicians are learning integrative techniques. While some may doubt the efficacy of natural, holistic medicine, its safety has been well established with many decades of experienced clinicians. When compared to the numerous side effects and potentially severe, even fatal, reactions to various medications, integrative medicine often offers a safer approach to health care that works."

—Dr. Bob Sears, pediatrician and author of *The Portable Pediatrician*

That first child sure is exciting. It's life changing when a baby enters the mix. Sure there's sleep deprivation, but one little smile makes it all worthwhile.

Then again, becoming a parent stimulates your worry gene. Suddenly every cough, rash, whimper, bruise, and pain sends you running to the pediatrician. While Dr. Rosen would be happy to see you in his office, many treatments can be initiated at home. This chapter is designed to highlight the most common baby ailments you'll face.

Colic

It's one thing to have a crybaby; it's quite another to have an inconsolable baby. Colic is estimated to affect at least one out of every five babies and is marked by the rule of threes: inconsolable crying for at least three hours a day, three days a week, for at least three weeks' duration. Theories abound on the cause, but doctors now think that the babies' nervous systems are not fully developed and some may become overstimulated by normal sights, sounds, and smells. Sometimes these babies need an extra month or two to adjust to life outside the uterus. Doctors also speculate that colic may be related to food sensitivities or a disturbance of intestinal bacteria.

According to Harvey Karp, MD, author of *The Happiest Baby on the Block*, colic is a serious problem. Dr. Karp suggests the key to understanding colic lies in the differences between the environments in and out of the womb and that babies are born before they're ready for the abrupt change.

> "In the womb, they enjoy a non-stop symphony of sensations: Touch, jiggly motion and the non-stop whoosh of the blood flow (louder than a vacuum cleaner ... 24/7). So, to our babies, being placed alone in a dark, quiet room creates massive sensory deprivation. Some kids fall apart without the womb rhythms. However, when you correctly imitate the womb sensations, it literally turns on an inborn calming reflex. As with any reflex, it can only be turned on with simple, but precise actions. The five specific steps that imitate the womb and turn on the "calming reflex" are the "5 S's" of swaddling, the side or stomach position, shushing, swinging or tiny jiggling motion, and sucking."

The never-ending crying is the most common sign of a colicky baby. Other symptoms include irregular sleeping habits, gas, clenched fists, and general irritability.

If you're at your wit's end with a crying baby, consider these conventional and alternative treatment options before your patience disappears.

Colic Treatment Alternatives: Side-by-Side Comparison

	Conventional Remedy	Treatment Alternative
Generic Treatment	Simethicone	Chamomile Tea
Sample Brand Name Treatment	Mylicon Infant Drops	Traditional Medicinals Organic Chamomile Tea
How it works	Helps break up gas bubbles in the abdomen, reducing bloating and discomfort	Contains natural chemicals that help relax a baby's intestinal tract and nervous system
Dosage	Under 2 years and under 24 lbs: 0.3mL up to 12 doses per day; Over 2 years and over 24 lbs: 0.6mL up to 12 doses per day	1 oz up to three times per day
Active Ingredients	Simethicone	Organic chamomile flower
Common Mild Side Effects	None	None
Less Common Serious Side Effects	Allergic reaction (rash, hives, swelling, itching, trouble breathing)	Allergic reaction (hives, itching, trouble breathing, dizziness, chest tightness)

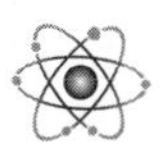

Science Says

The Department of Pediatrics at the Italian Universita di Torino studied the effectiveness of an extract of chamomile, fennel, and lemon balm in breast-fed colicky infants. Ninety-three infants were given either a placebo or the phytotherapeutic agent twice a day for one week. Crying time reduction was observed in 85 percent of babies given the herbal extract versus just 49 percent of those getting the placebo.

Natural Selection

If chamomile tea doesn't do the job, consider olive oil. Rubbing warm olive oil on your baby's belly in a circular motion as part of an infant massage routine may help soothe and relax him. You can also try adding a teaspoon of fennel seeds to boiling water, then serving this fennel tea, cooled to lukewarm, to your baby.

Cradle Cap

If only cradle cap referred to fashionable baby headgear worn in the crib. Babies everywhere could crawl the catwalk showing off their trendy cradle caps. It could become a billion-dollar industry.

Unfortunately, cradle cap is anything but fashionable. It's patchy, yellow, flaky skin most commonly seen on a baby's scalp. Cradle cap is also known to drift down to the eyebrows, forehead, and ears.

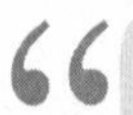

Parental Guidance

"We've always found good success with olive oil for cradle cap. I put olive oil on my baby's head, wait 15 minutes, and then take off any flakes with one of those lice nit combs. Then I give the baby a shampoo, and after washing the shampoo out and drying off the baby's head, I comb out any residual scabs. I wait another week or so and do it again. The longer you let the olive oil stay on, the less it seems to hurt the baby when you use the comb."

—Carmiya, mom to three young kids

According to popular myths, cradle cap can be caused by bacterial infections, allergies, or poor hygiene. In fact, doctors aren't in agreement on the true cause of cradle cap. The two most common theories are fungal infections and overactive sebaceous glands.

While not a serious condition, there's certainly nothing wrong with striving to give your offspring that baby-soft, flake-free skin back. Here's a look at the most common conventional and alternative treatment options available.

Cradle Cap Treatment Alternatives: Side-by-Side Comparison

	Conventional Remedy	Treatment Alternative
Generic Treatment	Mineral Oil	Olive Oil
Sample Brand Name Treatment	Johnson's Baby Oil	Spectrum Organic Extra Virgin Olive Oil
How it works	Helps loosen dead skin cells when applied to the scalp which can be combed out to remove flakes	Loosens dry flakes, which can be combed out; helps discourage fungal growth which may lead to cradle cap
Dosage	Cover affected area	Cover affected area
Active Ingredients	Mineral oil, fragrance	100% organic first cold pressed extra virgin unrefined Arbequina olive oil
Common Mild Side Effects	None	None
Less Common Serious Side Effects	Allergic reaction could cause skin rash	Allergic reaction could cause rash or itchy skin

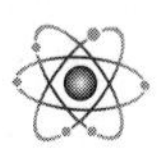

Science Says

The Department of Botany at Cairo University in Egypt studied the antifungal activity of olive oil. The olive oil compounds led to a significant reduction in amylase, lipase, keratinase, and urease enzyme activities for all tested fungal species, including *Candida albicans, Microsporum canis,* and *Trichophyton rubrum.*

Natural Selection

Aloe gel helps soothe and moisturize a baby's dry scalp. Also, shampooing your baby's hair with shampoos containing coconut oil or tea tree oil will help reduce flakes.

Diaper Rash

Diapers serve an important role in babyhood. They contain waste rather than deposit it on your sofa, in the car, and around the house. We're all thankful for the invention of diapers.

Unfortunately, the term *diaper* has also been linked to the most famous of baby rashes: diaper rash. The most common causes include:

- Wipes and creams with ingredients that irritate your baby's bottom
- Changes in stool consistency, which has various causes (including teething or the introduction of new foods)
- Too much time spent in dirty diapers, leading to skin irritation

The warm and moist nature of your baby's bottom doesn't help matters. It becomes a breeding ground for yeast and bacteria, which can also lead to diaper rash. However it comes about, you'll notice red, irritated, or bumpy skin on your baby's bottom, thighs, and genitals.

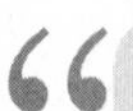

Parental Guidance

"My favorite natural remedy is calendula cream. I've seen amazing results on eczema and diaper rash with my son, as well as rapid healing of scrapes and cuts."

—Robyn, mother to a 2-year-old boy

When diaper rash gets really uncomfortable, your baby is likely to resist diaper changes. Maybe he knows the wiping is going to be anything but a good time. Your best bet is to wipe out that rash as soon as possible with one of these conventional or natural treatment alternatives.

Diaper Rash Treatment Alternatives: Side-by-Side Comparison

	Conventional Remedy	Treatment Alternative
Generic Treatment	Zinc oxide (with other ingredients)	Calendula
Sample Brand Name Treatment	Balmex Diaper Rash Cream	California Baby Calendula Cream
How it works	Soothes irritated skin and provides protective layer on skin to prevent future irritation	Soothes and heals dry or damaged skin as affected areas absorb the cream
Dosage	Apply cream liberally and promptly after each diaper change.	Apply cream to affected areas several times per day.
Active Ingredients	Zinc Oxide	Calendula flower
Common Mild Side Effects	None	None
Less Common Serious Side Effects	Allergic reaction	Allergic reaction

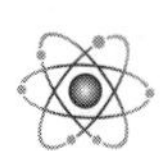

Science Says

The Department of Biochemistry at the Amala Cancer Research Center in Kerala, India, studied the wound-healing effectiveness of flower extract of *calendula officinalis.* After eight days, the group treated with calendula extract achieved 90 percent wound closure while the control group only showed 51 percent wound closure.

Natural Selection

Beyond calendula cream, applying a little cornstarch to the baby's bottom will help keep the area dry and reduce friction. Also consider a bath with oatmeal flakes (i.e., Aveeno brand) to soothe irritated skin. Finally, there's nothing like a little naked time to air out the rash (keep your little one off the sofa and carpets for this one). When in doubt, air it out!

Newborn Eye Discharge (Blocked Tear Ducts)

Babies' eyes draw us in. There's something about those big, staring blues, browns, and hazels that melt parents worldwide. It's no wonder we're concerned when a blocked tear duct strikes. Anything that messes with one of our baby's best assets is sure to rattle some parental nerves.

Blocked tear ducts occur when the nasolacrimal duct is obstructed. This prevents tears from easily draining from the eye to the nasal passage as they normally do. With baby tear ducts so small in size, it's no surprise they can become blocked so easily.

Spotting a blocked tear duct is not always easy; you may simply be dealing with an eyelash or dirt in the eye. However, if you see watery eyes; excessive tearing; or a clear or yellow discharge, then it's likely to be a blocked duct.

If your baby has a blocked tear duct, you should consider one of these conventional or natural treatment options to bring back those beautiful baby browns (or blues, or hazels)

Eye Discharge Treatment Alternatives: Side-by-Side Comparison

	Conventional Remedy	Treatment Alternative
Generic Treatment	Erythromycin	Breast milk
Sample Brand Name Treatment	E-Mycin Ointment	None
How it works	Helps decrease bacterial cell growth and hinder further development	Helps lubricate affected area and has antimicrobial properties that fight infection
Dosage	Clean affected area and apply ointment three times per day.	Put breast milk drops on finger and let it drip into corner of affected eye up to six times day.
Active Ingredients	Erythromycin, petrolatum, mineral oil	Protein, fat, carbohydrates, minerals
Common Mild Side Effects	Skin irritation, redness	None
Less Common Serious Side Effects	Allergic reaction	None

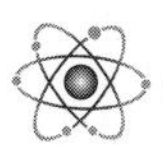

Science Says

The Journal of Tropical Pediatrics published a study of the effectiveness of switching from antibiotic eye drops to mother's milk drops as a treatment for duct obstruction. The study describes anti-inflammatory characteristics and antibacterial activity associated with mother's milk. Good to know if you're stuck in the tropics with a baby with a blocked tear duct.

Natural Selection

Applying a cotton ball soaked in warm water or warm chamomile tea to the blocked duct(s) and massaging gently in a clockwise direction several times a day can clear eye discharge and help open up the duct. Optique-1 eye drops by Boiron, a homeopathic solution, may also offer quick relief.

Spitting Up (Baby Reflux)

Just about anything a baby does is cute. Cooing, rolling over, sitting up, smiling, and waving all make parenting worthwhile. On the flip side, spitting up is more of a parental rite of passage. Ruining your nicest button-down with today's breakfast is your ticket to the parental club.

Spitting up, or baby reflux, is the regurgitation of food or milk soon after ingestion. In most cases, spitting up occurs while feeding or during the post-feed burping.

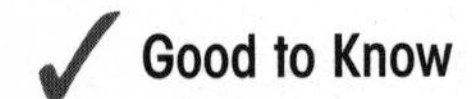

Baby reflux is most prevalent in babies 1 to 4 months of age and usually resolves spontaneously by 6 to 12 months. Up to 65 percent of healthy infants spit up or regurgitate from time to time, but this percentage drops to 1 percent by age 1.

The valve between the esophagus and stomach helps keep food down after eating or drinking. In babies, this valve is not yet fully developed. This leads to regurgitation, especially if too much food is consumed or too much air is swallowed.

If you're losing your shirt thanks to a regurgitating baby, you'll want to carefully consider these treatment options. Your dry cleaning bill just may depend on it.

Spitting Up Treatment Alternatives: Side-by-Side Comparison

	Conventional Remedy	Treatment Alternative
Generic Treatment	Ranitidine	Dairy elimination
Sample Brand Name Treatment	Zantac	None
How it works	Helps reduce stomach acid and aid in the easy digestion of food and milk	Removing dairy from the baby's diet (i.e., cow's milk) or a breastfeeding mom's diet can reduce instances of reflux due to cow's milk allergy or sensitivity.
Dosage	Take 1 mL two times per day and check with doctor for any changes based on age and weight of child.	Not applicable
Active Ingredients	Ranitidine	Not applicable
Common Mild Side Effects	Headache, fatigue, dizziness, diarrhea, constipation, sleep disruption	Possible vitamin D or calcium deficiency if these needs are not otherwise met
Less Common Serious Side Effects	Fever, nausea, change in heart rate, vision problems, chest pain, bruising, jaundice	None

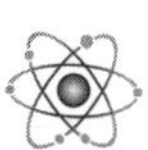

Science Says

The Pediatric GI Division at the Babies' Hospital in Palermo, Italy, studied milk-induced reflux in infants less than 1 year of age. Researchers found cow's milk allergy and gastroesophageal reflux (GER) to be among the most common disturbances in infants and recommended pediatricians screen for possible cow's milk allergies in all infants with GER.

Natural Selection

It's best to keep your baby upright after feedings for at least 20-30 minutes. This helps the food and drink flow more smoothly from the esophagus into the stomach—and stay there. Babies with GER also tend to spit up less when fed smaller amounts more frequently. Consider BPA-free baby bottles designed to minimize air bubbles during drinking. And keep in mind this advice from noted natural birth and lactation specialist Debra Pascali-Bonaro, LCCE, BDT/PDT (www.motherlovedoulas.com): "With the many short and long term health benefits of breastfeeding, especially for a baby's developing immune system, breastfeeding is the perfect opportunity to offer your baby the best beginning."

Teething

Teeth sure are fascinating. What other body part are we born without? Furthermore, what other body part falls out only to regrow bigger? Could you imagine if the same thing happened with your tongue, arms, or eyes? Growing up sure would be more interesting.

Turns out teeth have the unique distinction of appearing after birth. It's a nice system for newborns, who really don't need teeth at the outset. Unfortunately, the process of growing that first batch is not the most comfortable experience.

Teething occurs when a baby's primary teeth start to break through the gums. This typically begins when a baby is between 5 and 9 months of age and continues until all 20 teeth appear.

The most common teething symptoms include excessive drooling, swollen gums, irritability, and slight fever. Of course, parents' least favorite symptom, sleeplessness, often joins the party. When you first notice teeth breaking through the gums, be sure to read this section on conventional and natural treatment alternatives to soothe the effects of building a smile.

Parental Guidance

"For teething we try to avoid over-the-counter remedies for pain management. Since our son was three weeks old, he has worn a Baltic amber necklace to alleviate teething pain. We know it works, because on the few occasions that he was not wearing it, he was a miserable mess. We've only had to administer pain reliever two or three times in his entire life, and that was when he was cutting molars."

—Christine, mother to a 2-year-old boy

Teething Treatment Alternatives: Side-by-Side Comparison

	Conventional Remedy	Treatment Alternative
Generic Treatment	Benzocaine	*Chamomilla*
Sample Brand Name Treatment	Baby Orajel	Boiron Camilia
How it works	Provides temporary relief of sore gums associated with teething	Provides natural relief from painful gums and irritability associated with teething
Dosage	Under 4 months: consult a doctor before usage; over 4 months: apply pea-sized amount to area up to four times daily	Under 1 month: do not use; over 1 month: squeeze entire contents of single-use dose into mouth and repeat two more times every 15 minutes as needed
Active Ingredients	Benzocaine	*Chamomilla vulgaris* 9c, *phytolacca decandra* 5c, *Rheum officinale* 5c
Common Mild Side Effects	Swelling, rash, fever	None
Less Common Serious Side Effects	Methemoglobinemia, a blood disorder causing too little oxygen in red blood cells	None

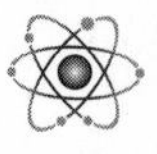

Science Says

Researchers at Case Western Reserve University in Cleveland, Ohio, found that chamomile blocks nitrous oxide production, an inflammation marker, explaining how chamomile and its derivatives work as effective anti-inflammatory agents.

Natural Selection

Babies sure do like to chew on things. Consider placing a teething ring or a wet washcloth in the freezer then serving it to your little one. Look for teething toys free of BPA and other harmful plasticizers. Mesh feeders containing frozen fruits or vegetables also help soothe and numb gums.

Thrush

If you asked me back in college about thrush, I would've assumed you were talking about a new rock band. I'd have expected to see them touring college campuses while young adults rocked out to their latest single.

It's amazing how parenthood changes your perspective. I now understand thrush to be a yeast infection that develops in the mouth, typically on the tongue, inner cheeks, or throat. I guess it's not the catchiest name for a rock band after all.

While yeast is present in all digestive systems, an overabundance of yeast may be attributed to hormones shifting just after birth. That could explain why thrush is most common in babies two months and younger.

Thrush typically manifests as white lesions on the inside of a baby's mouth, usually on the tongue, gums, and insides of the cheeks. You'll notice a cottage cheese-like texture or appearance to these lesions.

Unlike milk deposits, they don't scrape off easily. The discomfort from thrush can make even the best eater resist breast- or bottle-feeding. Consider these treatment alternatives at the first sign of thrush.

Thrush Treatment Alternatives: Side-by-Side Comparison

	Conventional Remedy	Treatment Alternative
Generic Treatment	Nystatin	Probiotics
Sample Brand Name Treatment	Bio-Statin	Klaire Infant Ther-Biotic Complete
How it works	The antifungal medicine weakens the membranes of the infected cells.	Helps inhibit the growth of infected cells and supports the body's immune system
Dosage	Less than 30 days old: 0.5mL applied to each side of mouth four times per day; More than 30 days old: 1.0mL applied to each side of mouth four times per day	¼ teaspoon taken daily with food or drink
Active Ingredients	Nystatin	*Lactobacillus, Bifidobacterium,* inulin
Common Mild Side Effects	Nausea, upset stomach, vomiting, diarrhea	None
Less Common Serious Side Effects	Allergic reaction	Allergic reaction, diarrhea

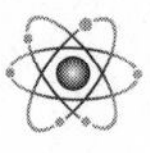

Science Says

The Department of Odontology at Umea University in Sweden studied the role probiotics play in oral health. Eight probiotic strains were tested for growth inhibition of the yeast *Candida*, a common cause of thrush. *Lactobacilli* probiotics significantly thwarted the growth of *Candida.*

Natural Selection

Infants over six months old not sensitive to dairy can try organic yogurts or other cultured foods like kefir. These cultured foods contain natural probiotics—consider dipping your finger in yogurt then targeting the affected area in your child's mouth. Not a yogurt fan, or dairy sensitive? Pure virgin coconut oil applied inside the baby's mouth can decrease bacteria and help prevent additional infected cells from developing.

Umbilical Cord Care

"Would you like to cut the cord, Daddy?" It's a common question asked in delivery rooms around the world. The simple snip detaches your baby from its prenatal lifeline of nutrients and oxygen to support growth in the womb.

The umbilical cord is usually clamped when it's cut, and then it naturally falls off after about one to three weeks. In the meantime, it's important to keep the area clean and dry. This is the best way to prevent any unwanted infections from developing.

You'll notice the umbilical cord changing color as it prepares to fall off. It generally changes from green to brown to black in color. You may also notice an odor present just before the stump falls off. This stems from the dead tissue and cells associated with the umbilical cord. The belly button is then formed when the cord stump officially falls off.

✓ Good to Know

Every time a new baby is born, the parents have a once-in-a-lifetime opportunity to save the baby's cord blood stem cells for possible future medical uses. Cord blood stem cells have been used to treat many life-threatening diseases such as leukemia and certain types of cancers. Researchers hope to one day extend cord blood usage to treat currently incurable conditions such as brain injuries and juvenile diabetes.

The following simple conventional and alternative treatment options can ensure an infection-free umbilical cord stump experience for parents.

Umbilical Cord Treatment Alternatives: Side-by-Side Comparison

	Conventional Remedy	Treatment Alternative
Generic Treatment	Rubbing Alcohol	Air
Sample Brand Name Treatment	Swan Rubbing Alcohol	None
How it works	Expedites process of drying out umbilical cord area and staves off infection	Exposure to air helps dry out area safely and quickly until cord falls off naturally.
Dosage	Swab umbilical cord with alcohol during diaper changes	Not applicable
Active Ingredients	Isopropyl alcohol, water	Not applicable
Common Mild Side Effects	Irritation or redness of the skin	None
Less Common Serious Side Effects	Skin infection	None

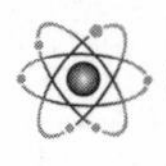

Science Says

Researchers in Ontario, Canada, studied alcohol versus natural drying for newborn umbilical cord care. More than 1,800 newborns were observed from birth until separation of the cord. Half received isopropyl alcohol at each diaper change and the other half air-dried naturally. There was no difference in the development of cord infections for either test group. Scientists concluded, "Evidence does not support continued use of alcohol for newborn cord care."

Natural Selection

For umbilical cords developing some bacterial overgrowth, witch hazel (extract of the bark or leaf of the *Hamamelis* plant), is a topically applied astringent that can speed up the drying process. Covering the cord stump with sterilized gauze will help keep the area dry and secure while your baby wears a diaper.

Spotlight On: Infant Massage

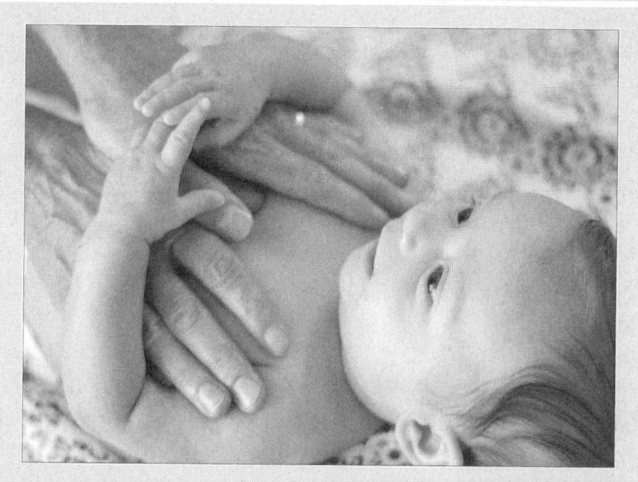

Infant massage has many proven benefits.

How would you like to help your baby both grow and feel better? Increasing evidence points to these outcomes when babies are on the receiving end of a gentle, caressing touch. Infant massage is a skin-to-skin connection between parent and baby that creates powerful attachment and connection without a single word.

Researchers are discovering a plethora of infant massage benefits even beyond baby growth and behavior. It may actually promote better sleeping; relieve colic symptoms; and even enhance an infant's motor skills, intellectual development, and immune system.

Infant massage has proven to be exceptionally effective for preterm infants. In various scientific studies, preterm infants receiving regular massage gained significantly more weight and experienced increased bone density compared to untreated infants.

So how exactly do you reap all these benefits for your little one? Simply take a comfy blanket or towel and a massage oil you know your baby can tolerate. It's worth testing the oil on a small spot on your baby's skin to check for allergic reactions the day before the first massage. Grapeseed or sesame seed oil are commonly used. The best time to massage is when your baby is in a quiet, alert state. This is most common post-feeding or pre-nap time.

Sit on the floor with the soles of your feet touching in a diamond shape and drape a blanket over your feet. Now you can lay your baby down and cradle her head with your feet. Begin the massage section by section, spending less or more time in each area depending on the reaction of your child. For more information on infant massage, check out the International Loving Touch Foundation (www.lovingtouch.com) or the Touch Research Institute at the University of Miami (www6.miami.edu/touch-research).

2

Watch Your Mouth

"To become educated holistically on behalf of your children is a tremendous gift. This knowledge brings you closer to the confidence that parenting needs, closer to the health and life you deserve, and closer to your children. The time and effort we have put into learning to parent holistically has been tremendously beneficial to our family. I support any efforts parents can make to learn more about how this approach to life and health can simplify your life, reduce the costs of healthcare, and benefit the relationships in your family."

—Mayim Bialik, PhD, actress in *The Big Bang Theory,* neuroscientist, holistic mom, and celebrity spokesperson for the Holistic Moms Network

"Watch your mouth" usually means a bar of soap is imminent for inappropriate language. Not the case in this chapter. Instead, we're talking about ailments appearing in your child's mouth. From cavities and cold sores to Coxsackie virus and sore throat, welcome to one-stop shopping for conventional and natural oral treatment alternatives.

Maybe this chapter will actually put a positive spin on the "watch your mouth" phrase. It could go from a parental threat to an oral hygiene and health savior.

Bad Breath

It's easy to only think of bad breath as a first date deal breaker. After all, who wants to lean in for that romantic moment only to whiff onion glaze from your date's steak tartar? However, bad breath can strike kids, too, from toddlers to teenagers. From play dates to hanging out after school, nobody wants their kid to inherit a reputation for stinky breath.

Medically known as halitosis, bad breath is best described as an unpleasant odor emitted from the mouth. While most consumed food enters the digestive tract, some food particles remain in the teeth and gums and on the tongue. As those food particles decompose, bad breath often results. Sleeping also leads to halitosis due to decreased saliva production.

Assuming you want your child to have minty fresh breath from conception through college, here's a look at conventional treatment and alternatives for combating bad breath.

Bad Breath Treatment Alternatives: Side-by-Side Comparison

	Conventional Remedy	Treatment Alternative
Generic Treatment	Antiseptic mouthwash	Probiotics
Sample Brand Name Treatment	Listerine Zero Clean Mint mouthwash	Klaire Ther-Biotic Complete Chewables
How it works	Helps kill germs, eliminate bacteria, and reduce food particles linked to bad breath	Contains probiotics that eradicate mouth germs and xylitol, a natural sugar alcohol that reduces bacteria growth

	Conventional Remedy	Treatment Alternative
Dosage	Over 6 years: rinse twice a day with 2/3 fluid ounce or 20mL (4 teaspoonfuls) for 30 seconds; do not swallow; Under 6 years: do not use	Over 2 years: chew 1-2 tablets per day 30-60 minutes after a meal
Active Ingredients	Water, sorbitol solution, propylene glycol, sodium lauryl sulfate, benzoic acid, sodium benzoate, poloxamer 407, sodium saccharin, flavor, sucralose, FD&C green no. 3	Probiotic blend of 25 billion CFU of *Lactobacilli* and *Bifidobacteria*, xylitol, inulin
Common Mild Side Effects	Potential discoloration of teeth	None
Less Common Serious Side Effects	None	Bloating, diarrhea

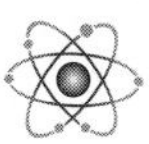

Science Says

Fukuoka Dental College in Japan studied the effects of probiotics on halitosis and oral health. Twenty patients with genuine halitosis were given *Lactobacillus salivarius* (a probiotic) and xylitol in tablet form daily. Not only did these patients see an improvement in their halitosis condition but they also showed reduced bleeding from periodontal pocket probing.

Natural Selection

Consider these additional treatment alternatives to battle bad breath:

- Many yogurts contain probiotics that help discourage the bacteria growth that leads to bad breath.
- Parsley contains chlorophyll, a natural breath cleanser when consumed.
- Natural herbs and spices such as anise, cloves, and fennel can disguise bad breath.

Canker Sores and Cold Sores

Next weekend is the big homecoming dance. Your teenage daughter should be basking in the glory of a high school rite of passage. Instead she's cowering in the bathroom, devastated by a cold sore on her lower lip. She's threatening never to leave the bathroom again, so parental job one is to cure that blemish pronto. Your daughter's high school legacy just might depend on choosing the right treatment plan.

Cold sores, also called fever blisters, are caused by the herpes simplex virus (HSV). The virus enters your child's body through a skin break inside or around her mouth. It's typically spread by sharing utensils, kissing an infected person, or even touching their saliva. The resulting red, swollen blisters can break open, leak fluid, and ultimately scab over in a few days.

Unlike cold sores, the cause of canker sores is unknown but researchers suspect a combination of these factors may lead to outbreaks:

- A minor injury to the mouth from a cheek bite or overly aggressive brushing
- Food allergies and sensitivities, particularly to eggs, nuts, cheese, and highly acidic food

- Nutritional deficiencies from diets lacking in zinc, iron, folic acid, and/or vitamin B_{12}
- An immune system defect that attacks healthy mouth cells instead of viruses and bacteria
- Celiac disease, an intestinal disorder caused by gluten sensitivity

While it's easy to confuse canker and cold sores inside the mouth, there's a major distinction. While canker sores are not contagious, cold sores are extremely contagious. Your child's best bet is to steer clear of saliva from and sharing utensils with a potentially infected person. In other words, fork-sharing on toddler play dates may not be your best decision.

Parental Guidance

"For canker sores, we use ¼ teaspoon turmeric and two teaspoons raw honey mixed together, and then apply it with a cotton swab on the spot. Burns for a moment, but feels better later."

—Carmiya, mom to three young kids

Even though canker sores and cold sores are different, the treatment typically is the same. Let's compare the two and dig a little deeper into natural alternatives.

Cold/Canker Sores Treatment Alternatives: Side-by-Side Comparison

	Conventional Remedy	Treatment Alternative
Generic Treatment	Camphor, menthol, and phenol	L-lysine
Sample Brand Name Treatment	Blistex medicated lip ointment	Super Lysine+
How it works	Medication relieves sore area and speeds healing time.	Cream applied to infected area soothes discomfort and shortens sore cycle time.
Dosage	Apply liberally to affected area.	Apply liberally to affected area.
Active Ingredients	Dimethicone, camphor menthol, phenol	L-lysine, flower extract, zinc oxide, tea tree oil
Common Mild Side Effects	Burning, stinging, redness, tingling	Tingling, burning
Less Common Serious Side Effects	Allergic reaction	None

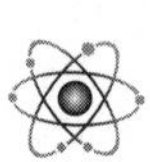

Science Says

USC Health Sciences conducted a study on the safety and effectiveness of lysine with botanicals and other nutrients in the treatment of herpes simplex virus. By the third day of treatment, 40 percent of study participants were healed, and 87 percent were healed by the sixth day. Conventional remedies typically offer similar healing cycle times; cold sores left untreated can last up to three weeks.

Natural Selection

When it comes to treating canker and cold sores, Super Lysine+ is not the only natural choice. From a homeopathic perspective, consider Traumeel drops. When applied several times per day and before sleep, the drops can relieve sore blisters and help them heal quicker. Your child will feel an initial sting but it will soon begin to soothe the tingling and irritation.

Cavities

If only your child fully understood the correlation between poor brushing habits and cavities. Nighttime routines sure would go smoother if children knew skipping the toothbrush could lead to a date with the dentist's drill. Somehow this logic fails to motivate 5-year-olds.

Cavities develop from the bacteria inside the mouth that feeds on food particles left behind after eating and drinking. Mixed together, lactic acid forms and ultimately decomposes the tooth enamel.

A cavity may be accompanied by a number of symptoms for your child. Sensitivity to hot or cold foods and beverages is often an early indicator. A throbbing feeling in the tooth is another sign. A visit to the pediatric dentist will be the only surefire way to know if a cavity is present.

Assuming your child would prefer to avoid dates with the drill, let's check out cavity prevention options and keep dentist visits to simple cleanings.

Cavities Treatment Alternatives: Side-by-Side Comparison

	Conventional Remedy	Treatment Alternative
Generic Treatment	Fluoride vitamins	Xylitol
Sample Brand Name Treatment	Luride (chewable tablets)	Spry Oral Rinse
How it works	Contains a mineral that strengthens teeth and reduces tooth decay risk caused by acid and food bacteria	Bacteria cannot break down xylitol into lactic acid; xylitol helps prevent the bacteria from adhering to the enamel.
Dosage	Over six months: take one tablet per day with or without food	When child is old enough to swish, use for 30 seconds in mouth.
Active Ingredients	Sodium fluoride	Xylitol
Common Mild Side Effects	Staining of teeth	None
Less Common Serious Side Effects	Diarrhea, hives, rash, seizures, trembling, stomach discomfort, unusual increase in saliva, vomiting	Gas, diarrhea

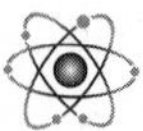

Science Says

The University of Washington School of Dentistry in Seattle, Washington, studied the effectiveness of xylitol in children age 9 to 15 months. The primary goal was to determine the effectiveness of xylitol in preventing tooth decay in the primary teeth of very young children. In the study, 100 children received either xylitol or a control syrup two to three times daily. Researchers determined a total daily dose of 8 grams was effective in preventing early childhood tooth decay.

Natural Selection

Xylitol is one treatment alternative to battle back against cavities. You can also consider increasing calcium in your child's diet as it helps protect tooth enamel. Weston A. Price was a prominent dentist in the early 1900s who explored and publicized the relationship between nutrition and dental health. He is often cited as the father of holistic dentistry. Additionally, sage is known to have antibacterial elements that help prevent cavities; it can be mixed with water and baking soda as a natural toothpaste. Arrowroot powder, made from the *Maranta arundinacea* plant, was initially used by Native Americans and West Indian peoples as a natural tooth cleanser. It turns out this botanical does have antibacterial properties and can be applied like sage, with water and baking soda as a paste.

Coxsackie Virus

If you've ever heard of hand, foot, and mouth disease, then you might be curious about its causes—the curiously-named Coxsackie virus. Dr. Gilbert Dalldorf coined the name based on his work in the 1940s in Coxsackie, New York, a small town on the Hudson River. Most common in children between 6 months and 3 years of age, this is a highly contagious virus that can also infect older children.

The first sign of the Coxsackie virus is usually small, white or red sores on the lips, gums, throat, or inner cheek of a child's mouth. From there, these often-painful sores are frequently accompanied by the following symptoms:

- Excessive drooling
- Fever and fussiness
- Rashes on the hands and feet
- Reduced appetite and refusal to eat or drink due to mouth pain

While flu season usually winds down in the spring, the Coxsackie virus peaks in summer and autumn. Year-round outbreaks are common in tropical climates.

Although they typically last one week, the Coxsackie virus sores can be combated sooner with available conventional and alternative treatments.

Coxsackie Virus Treatment Alternatives: Side-by-Side Comparison

	Conventional Remedy	Treatment Alternative
Generic Treatment	Aluminum/magnesium antacid (Maalox), Diphenhydramine (Benadryl), viscous lidocaine (xylocaine)	Homeopathic blend
Sample Brand Name Treatment	Maalox, Benadryl, xylocaine	Traumeel-S (tablet)
How it works	The three medications together coat sores and topically provide only temporary relief.	The natural inflammatory contains botanical and mineral ingredients to provide relief from mouth sore pain.
Dosage	For children able to swish and spit, mix 1 tsp each of Maalox, Benadryl, and xylocaine and swish in the mouth; For children over 1 unable to swish, mix equal parts Maalox and Benadryl on the child's lips, tongue, and inner cheeks with a Q-tip.	Infants and children under 6 years of age: take ½ tablet 3 times per day; Over 6 years: take one tablet 3 times per day.

	Conventional Remedy	Treatment Alternative
Active Ingredients	Maalox: magnesium; Benadryl: Diphenhydramin; Xylocaine: Lidocaine Hydrochloride	*Aconitum napellus* 3X, *arnica montana* 3X, belladonna 4X, *bellis perennis* flower 2X, *calendula* flower 2X, *chamomilla* 3X, *echinacea angustifolia* 2X, *echinacea purpurea* 2X, *hamamelis virginiana* 2X, *hepar sulfuris calcareum* 8X, *hypericum perforatum* 3X, *mercurius solubilis* 8X, *millefolium* 3X, *symphytum officinale* 8X*H*
Common Mild Side Effects	Maalox: nausea, constipation, diarrhea, headache; Benadryl: fatigue, dry mouth, dizziness, headache; Xylocaine: decreased sensation in the mouth and throat	None
Less Common Serious Side Effects	Maalox: black stools, painful urination, vomiting; Benadryl: seizure, ringing in the ears, irregular heartbeat; Xylocaine: blurred vision, vomiting, irregular heartbeat, trembling	Allergic reaction

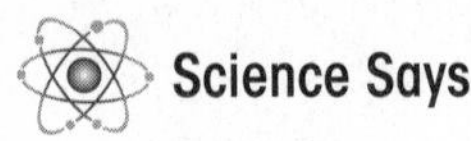

Science Says

Published clinical trials of Traumeel-S for mouth sores have been limited to the treatment of chemotherapy-induced stomatitis in children, but the studies are compelling. However, for kids older than one, the answer just may be cinnamon honey tea, a classic Ayurvedic remedy. Simply place two or three cinnamon sticks (cinnamon contains the chemical eugenol with known anesthetic properties) in boiling water for five minutes. Remove the sticks and add one tablespoon of honey (shown to have anti-inflammatory properties). Sipping 2 to 4 ounces 3 to 4 times per day just may soothe Coxsackie virus sores.

Natural Selection

Additional soothing and comfort measures can help your child handle the Coxsackie virus. For example, cool yogurts can help coat the sores to decrease discomfort. Garlic cloves, when soaked in and then removed from hot water, can be consumed for pain relief. Finally, zinc supplements help boost immunity and may proactively prevent the likelihood of a viral outbreak in your family.

Sore Throat

You just might take your throat for granted. After all, it quietly keeps the food you eat moving along to the digestive tract. Every so often, however, that scratchy feeling tells you a sore throat is on the horizon. For youngsters, it's typically not dangerous, but it's certainly a bothersome ailment.

Viral infections, such as the common cold and flu, can trigger sore throats. Bacterial infections, such as strep throat, can also lead to a sore throat. Even allergies, particularly the postnasal drip associated with mold, dust, and pollen allergies, can activate a sore throat.

That scratchy throat feeling is the most common symptom. Parents would likely add persistent kid complaining as another sore throat symptom. Before it turns into anything more serious, here are the conventional and natural choices for soothing your child's throat.

Parental Guidance

"My daughter suffers from a sore throat a few times each winter. It hurts her to talk, which is uncharacteristic for my wonderful chatterbox. All it takes is a couple of sprays of propolis echinacea, and the pain is gone. Propolis echinacea spray has been a lifesaver for us and travels with us wherever we go in the winter months. It is natural, safe, effective, and just requires getting used to the different taste."

—Tamra, mom to a 7-year-old daughter

Sore Throat Treatment Alternatives: Side-by-Side Comparison

	Conventional Remedy	Treatment Alternative
Generic Treatment	Benzocaine	Herbal tea
Sample Brand Name Treatment	Cepacol Fizzlers	Traditional Medicinals Organic Throat Coat Tea
How it works	Dissolves on the tongue to relieve sore throats	Soothes sore throat symptoms
Dosage	Under 5 years: don't use; over 5 years: let one tablet dissolve on tongue every 2 hours	One cup of tea as needed
Active Ingredients	Benzocaine	Licorice root, slippery elm bark, marshmallow root

	Conventional Remedy	Treatment Alternative
Common Mild Side Effects	Headache, confusion, fast heart rate, pale skin, feeling light-headed	None
Less Common Serious Side Effects	Oozing, blistering, severe burning, grey or bluish skin appearance	None

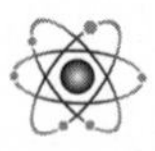

Science Says

Researchers in California studied the effectiveness of Throat Coat tea in a placebo-controlled trial.. They concluded, "Throat Coat is significantly superior to placebo and provided a rapid, temporary relief of sore throat pain in patients with pharyngitis." In another study, Indian scientists found that licorice root (an ingredient in Throat Coat tea) gargle was more effective than placebo for postoperative sore throats.

Persistent sore throats could be indicative of tonsillitis, a more severe condition. Look for additional symptoms such as swollen lymph nodes; difficulty swallowing; and red, swollen tonsils. Over 500,000 tonsillectomies are performed annually on U.S. children younger than 15 years. Before rushing to surgery—which has come under mainstream scrutiny—try gargling with salt water to alleviate early onset symptoms. In fact, the American Academy of Otolaryngology now recommends at least seven episodes of recurrent throat infection a year before undergoing a tonsillectomy.

Natural Selection

Grandparents far and wide have home remedies galore to improve sore throats. Among the most popular are ...

- Herbal teas with honey—sip as needed. Raspberry, sage, and turmeric are some of the more popular choices.
- Gargling—various concoctions have been time-tested for soothing throats. The most basic is warm water with salt, but other solutions include mixing water with apple cider vinegar, horseradish, or ginger.
- Vaporizers—cool mist can alleviate the hoarseness associated with sore throats.

Swollen Glands (Nodes)

Do you remember pop quizzes from grade school? Well here's one for you: can you point to your lymph nodes? If your hands are on your feet, guess again.

Lymph nodes are part of your immune system and are small nodules of tissue heavily concentrated around the throat, armpits, chest, and groin area. Many people think of them as swollen glands when, in fact, these nodes are part of the immune system.

Among all these lymph nodes, some are swollen more frequently than others, particularly under the jaw. There are several possible causes for swollen nodes including infection, virus, immune disorders, and even simple inflammation. Sore throat, stuffy nose, and fever may also accompany enlarged and tender lymph nodes.

The next time you feel that bulge under your child's jaw, consider these conventional and natural treatment options to reduce pain and discomfort.

Swollen Glands Treatment Alternatives: Side-by-Side Comparison

	Conventional Remedy	Treatment Alternative
Generic Treatment	Amoxicillin and clavulinic acid	Lymph massage
Sample Brand Name Treatment	Augmentin	None
How it works	Helps treat the bacterial infection by destroying the outer walls of the bacteria cells	Massage stimulates the flow of lymph, which helps filter foreign substances and fight infection.
Dosage	Under 88 lbs: consult a doctor for dosage; Over 88 lbs: 500mg every 12 hours or 250mg every 8 hours	Massage gently every few hours as needed
Active Ingredients	Amoxicillin	None
Common Mild Side Effects	Mild rash, diarrhea, unsettled stomach, vomiting	None
Less Common Serious Side Effects	Hives, severe rash, vaginal infection, difficulty breathing	Temporary and mild flu- like symptoms such as upset stomach, nausea, or slight fever

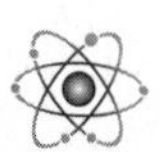

Science Says

Most data on lymph node swelling therapy comes from research on lymphedema, the severe congestion of lymph nodes and the skin and tissues surrounding the nodes. The Dermatology Department at the University of London in the United Kingdom published a review noting that massage is a key component in integrative lymphedema therapy by improving the drainage of excess fluid from congested tissues to normally draining lymph node areas.

Natural Selection

Essential oils, like lavender, can help soothe and decrease swelling in the lymph nodes when added to the massage routine. Many oils, like chamomile, also contain natural chemicals that counteract inflammation to help soothe swollen nodes.

Spotlight On: Probiotics

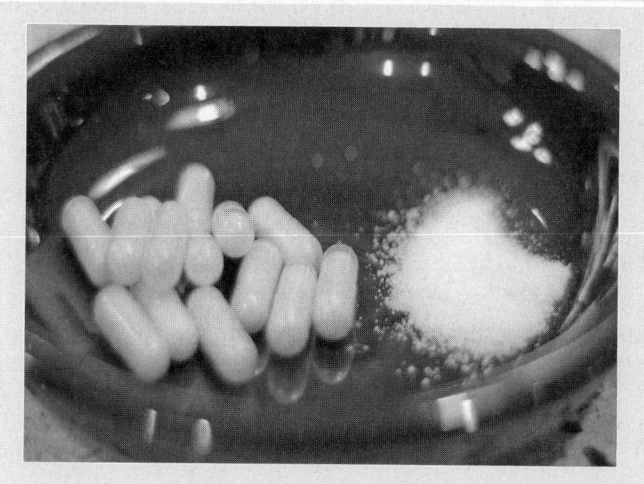

Probiotics in supplement form.

Literally meaning "for life," probiotics are defined by the World Health Organization as "live microorganisms which, when administered in adequate amounts, confer a health benefit on the host." There is increasing evidence that probiotics are helpful in treating and preventing a variety of ailments. The main rationale behind probiotic effectiveness is their ability to normalize intestinal microbial flora. These microorganisms, some classified as bacteria and some as yeast, have been demonstrated to have a positive effect on both digestive and immune function.

Many foods contain probiotics. The most well known is yogurt with active cultures, particularly *Lactobacillus* and *Bifidobacterium*. However, since an all-yogurt diet is unrealistic for your kid, and some are particularly dairy-sensitive, probiotic supplements are a welcome alternative to help normalize microbial flora.

A number of randomized controlled trials have tested the safety and effectiveness of probiotics across a wide range of infant and childhood ailments. These include infectious diarrhea, antibiotic-associated diarrhea, constipation, urinary tract infections, irritable bowel syndrome, Crohn's Disease, and atopic disorders like eczema and asthma. While more analysis is needed to fully confirm probiotic benefits for this entire scope of ailments, studies thus far do point toward positive outcomes.

The biggest benefit of probiotics may be their safety and ease of digestion for kids. Numerous clinical trials have shown minimal adverse reactions, and long-term usage appears to be safe and well tolerated, even in premature neonates. That all adds up to an excellent natural treatment alternative when you want to steer your kids clear of medications with potentially harmful side effects.

3

Seeing, Hearing, and Smelling

"The road to becoming a holistic parent is a journey. We learn from other parents and become aware of the vast array of natural healing options available to us over time and incorporate them into our daily lives when we discover not only how safe they are, but how well they work with the body to heal. Having natural remedies is a priority for many holistic moms, so that when those sniffles and coughs come along we know that effective, non-toxic help is near."

—Nancy Massotto, Founder & Executive Director, Holistic Moms Network (www.holisticmoms.org)

Life without your eyes, ears, and nose sure would be challenging. Maybe that's why your child instantly complains the moment one of her senses is compromised. From crusty eyes to ear pain to clogged noses, this chapter is all about seeing, hearing, and smelling ailments.

So if your child ever woke with pinkeye, a ringing in his ears, or a nose that's too stuffy or too runny, this is the chapter for you.

Conjunctivitis (Pinkeye)

There's nothing like a child waking up to another beautiful day only to find out his eyes are crusted shut. All your son wants to do is pop out of bed, slap on some clothes, and run downstairs for a delicious breakfast. Unfortunately, pinkeye has temporarily disturbed the all-important sense of sight.

As a loving parent this loss of sight is no laughing matter. Eyes are delicate. The last thing you ever want is to jeopardize the long-term vision of your child. That said, let's better understand the causes and symptoms of conjunctivitis.

The majority of pinkeye cases are caused by viral and bacterial eye infections. To a lesser extent, allergies, chemicals, and smoke fumes may trigger an onset.

Parental Guidance

"When I was pregnant with my second daughter, I ended up with conjunctivitis in both eyes. My older daughter was still nursing and she caught it too. She was constantly rubbing her eyes and was disturbed by all the discharge. I gave her Eyebright herbal solution to take internally. We also used the homeopathic remedy *Euphrasia*, taken orally and by dabbing a solution of it on her eyes. We saw an immediate improvement and her eyes continued to heal with each application."
—Bo, mother to Audrey, 4, and Elisa, 1

The most common symptoms include the following:

- Swollen or red eyes
- Itching or burning feeling in the eyes
- A sensation that something is in the eyes
- Draining from the eye or more tearing than usual

If your kid's eyes are stricken with conjunctivitis, you'll undoubtedly be anxious to de-crust her eyes quickly (not to mention a clean bill of health for school). Let's break down conventional versus natural treatment alternatives to bring out the whites in your loved one's pinkeye.

Conjunctivitis Treatment Alternatives: Side-by-Side Comparison

	Conventional Remedy	Treatment Alternative
Generic Treatment	Tobramycin ophthalmic	*Euphrasia officinalis*
Sample Brand Name Treatment	Tobrex solution	Optique 1 from Boiron
How it works	Stops the growth of bacterial eye infections	Reduces red, dry, itchy, and burning irritations
Dosage	Mild cases: 1-2 drops every 4 hours; moderate cases: 2 drops every hour	Snap off single use dose and instill 1-2 drops in eyes 2-6 times per day
Active Ingredients	Tobramycin	*Cineraria maritima* 6C, *Euphrasia officinalis* 4X, *Calendula officinalis* 4X, kali muriaticum 10X, calcarea fluorica 10X, magnesia carbonica 10X, Silicea 10X
Common Mild Side Effects	Eye burning, stinging, itching, redness, light sensitivity	None
Less Common Serious Side Effects	Blurred vision, eyelid swelling	None

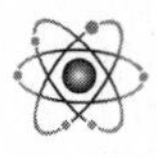

Science Says

Euphrasia is the key ingredient in Optique 1. Researchers at Witwatersand University in Johannesburg, South Africa, studied the effectiveness of *Euphrasia* single-dose eye drops in treating conjunctivitis. In the study, 12 general practitioners across Germany and Switzerland conducted tests on patients with inflammatory conjunctivitis. Each patient received single-dose eye drops one to five times per day as needed. Researchers discovered 82 percent of patients showed complete recovery while another 17 percent showed clear improvement.

Another common eye ailment is a stye in the eye. This bacterial infection typically causes a small, red lump along the edge of the eyelid. A warm, wet compress applied to the eye three to six times per day usually soothes and treats the stye. Conventionally, doctors may prescribe an antibiotic like erythromycin if the condition fails to respond to home-based remedies.

Natural Selection

Looking for even more natural choices to tackle pinkeye and get your child's eyesight clear again? Check out these two home remedies that just may get the job done:

- Damp tea bags—chamomile tea bags, heated then cooled, can be placed directly on irritated eyelids for soothing comfort.
- Breast milk—the most home-based of home-based remedies, can be applied directly to the infected eye(s). It's also safe for newborns.

Earache

Your little one tugs at his ear and you instantly think "Uh-oh, ear infection." But how do you really know if it's an earache, an ear infection, or just a silly ear-tugging gesture? This section and the next will cover the differences in causes, symptoms, and treatments for both earaches and ear infections. Let's start with earaches.

Ear pain in children is typically caused by a buildup of pressure from fluid in the middle ear space behind the eardrum. Your middle ear is connected to the nasal passages by the Eustachian tube. This tube plays an important function in your ear. It's responsible for allowing normal fluids to drain out of the middle ear while equalizing ear pressure. In young children, the Eustachian tube can be quite small and tortuous, making drainage difficult during times of congestion.

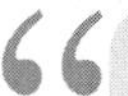

Parental Guidance

"Heat up a rice sock in the microwave. Then wrap it in cuddly fleece and encourage your child to rest the ouchie ear on it (use as pillow) until it cools."

—Roseanne, mother to Chris (age 16), Matt (age 14), and Alexandra (age 9)

Colds and allergies are the typical culprits in blocking the Eustachian tube from doing its job. The resulting pressure and inflammation causes the sensation of pain in the ear. Of course, an actual ear infection can cause similar pain, too. Many ear infections are, in fact, viral, though some can be caused by bacteria. If you're unsure why your child is in pain, your pediatrician has tools to figure this out. A quick look with an otoscope can rule out an infected eardrum as the cause of the ear pain. Assuming this time it's just an earache without an infection, let's break down the conventional versus natural treatment options.

Earache Treatment Alternatives: Side-by-Side Comparison

	Conventional Remedy	Treatment Alternative
Generic Treatment	Ibuprofen	Olive Oil
Sample Brand Name Treatment	Children's Advil Suspension	Spectrum Organic Olive Oil
How it works	Temporarily relieves minor aches and pains	Relieves earache pain when warmed and dropped into ear
Dosage	Under 2: ask a doctor; 2-3 years: 1 tsp 4 times per day; 4-5 years: 1½ tsp 6-8 years: 2 tsp 4 times per day; 9-10 years: 2½ tsp 4 times per day; over 11 years: 3 tsp 4 times per day	Small drops in affected ear every hour or two as needed 4 times per day
Active Ingredients	Ibuprofen	Olive oil
Common Mild Side Effects	Stomach pain, diarrhea, constipation, dizziness	None
Less Common Serious Side Effects	Allergic reaction	None

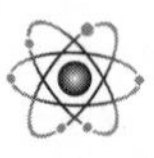

Science Says

According to the Natural Medicines Comprehensive Database, olive oil contains "oleocanthal, which might be responsible for some of the anti-inflammatory effects ... This compound shares some pharmacological properties with non-steroidal anti-inflammatory drugs (NSAIDs) such as ibuprofen."

Natural Selection

If you're not a fan of olive oil, you can achieve the same natural treatment objectives with sesame oil and a clove of garlic. Simply heat the sesame oil with the garlic clove crushed and mixed in. Then cool it to room temperature, enough to be safe to instill in your child's ear. Place a few drops of the garlic oil into the painful ear every four hours as needed for pain until the ache is gone.

Ear Infection

"Mommy, my ear hurts!" Your mind races. Did she bang her ear on the bedpost last night? Did she get water in there at bath time? Could it be an infection? You remember words of wisdom from your own parents to take ear pain seriously.

Two hours later, an ear infection is confirmed and you depart the pediatrician's office with an antibiotic prescription in hand. Driving home, you can't help but wonder if a more natural treatment could clear up this common infection.

Let's look at the symptoms and causes, as well as conventional versus natural treatment options, for dealing with those pesky ear infections.

Older children will more easily communicate their symptoms such as ear pain or earache, fullness in the ear, vomiting/diarrhea, and/or hearing loss in the affected ear.

If the Eustachian tubes, which connect the middle ears to the nose and throat, become blocked, fluid cannot adequately drain from the middle ear. This fluid then becomes the perfect breeding ground for viruses and bacteria, causing the eardrum to become inflamed and infected. The most common causes include ...

- Colds—upper respiratory viral infections, such as a cold or flu.
- Allergies—pollen, dust, food, and animal dander can all create the same effect as a cold.

- Environmental toxins—smoke, fumes, or other airborne toxins.
- Excess mucus and saliva—for babies, this buildup is common during teething.

✓ Good to Know

By age 2, more than 80 percent of children will experience at least one ear infection. The likely age range for ear infections is 6 months to 3 years of life. The most common ear infection, otitis media, is an inflammation and infection of the middle ear located just behind the eardrum.

Regardless of the symptoms or cause, you'll want to tackle an ear infection before it progresses to anything more serious. Here are both conventional and holistic ear infection treatment options.

Ear Infection Treatment Alternatives: Side-by-Side Comparison

	Conventional Remedy	Treatment Alternative
Generic Treatment	Antibiotic: amoxicillin	Garlic-mullein eardrops
Sample Brand Name Treatment	Amoxil	Herb Pharm Mullein Garlic
How it works	Amoxil is a penicillin antibiotic that fights bacteria in the body.	Inhibits or destroys germs present in the ear while controlling inflammation
Dosage	50 mg/kg per day in two divided doses	Place two or three drops into each ear every 4 hours as needed
Active Ingredients	Amoxicillin, synthetic antibiotic	A semi-mullein flower, garlic bulb, calendula flower

	Conventional Remedy	Treatment Alternative
Common Mild Side Effects	Stomach pain, nausea, vomiting, headache, or swollen, black, or "hairy" tongue	None
Less Common Serious Side Effects	White patches or sores inside mouth or on lips; numbness, pain, muscle weakness, severe tingling; fever, rash or itching; severe blisters, peeling, hives	Allergic reaction

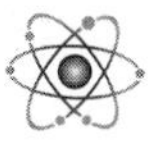

Science Says

The Pediatric and Adolescent Ambulatory Community Clinic at Tel Aviv University in Israel studied the effectiveness of herbal extracts (including garlic, mullein, and calendula) in the management of ear pain associated with ear infections. In this randomized and blind study, 103 children, ages 6-18, were given either a naturopathic extract or anesthetic eardrop (with or without amoxicillin). Researchers determined that children administered the naturopathic extract improved equally to those receiving a conventional anesthetic—and the children receiving the additional antibiotic showed no added improvement.

Natural Selection

As Amara Wagner, Certified Holistic Health Coach and owner of Amarawellness.com, states, "Garlic-mullein eardrops are incredibly effective and can be used not only for someone suffering with an ear infection, but also as a preventative measure. As with any other ailment, I take a holistic approach with my kids and clients and suggest that parents address the concern from several different angles including physical, emotional, and nutritional."

Herbal eardrops are not your only choice when it comes to treating pesky ear infections. A host of home remedies have been known to get the job done. With the American Academy of Pediatrics recommending against antibiotic use (when possible) for ear infections, any one of these could be a good bet:

- Massaging gently behind the ear and down the neck to aid in drainage
- Placing drops of hydrogen peroxide directly in each ear every four hours as needed
- Elevating your child's mattress when sleeping to help with drainage
- Inserting warm drops of either onion juice or olive oil directly in both ears

Runny Nose

Tissues are like fine china. You don't think about them much, but when you suddenly need some, you never have enough around. If your tissue budget just spiked, then one of your kids likely has a runny nose.

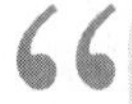

Parental Guidance

"One thing I always make a point of doing with my son when he has a sniffly cold is to wait until he's sleeping and then rub some vaseline on the outside of his nose (and a little into his nostrils). I do this each night that the cold lingers and it makes a huge difference with protecting the skin from getting sore and red."

—Jeanellen, mother to 2-year-old Ian

Mucus actually serves an important function in your nose. It keeps germs, dirt, and bacteria from marching into your lungs. However, when you get sick, your nose goes into mucus-making overtime to keep all the germs out of your body. It can start running down your throat, right out your nose, and (hopefully) into a tissue—or sleeve of an untrained toddler. Whether your runny nose stems from a cold or allergies, you'll want to find an effective treatment before your local drugstore runs out of tissues.

✓ Good to Know

Runny noses are not exclusive to the common cold. Allergies cause runny nose when you're exposed to the allergen. Tears from crying can mix with mucus and cause a runny nose. Cold days even cause runny noses. As your nose tries to warm up the cold air before passing it to your lungs, the extra blood flow required leads to extra mucus production.

Whether your runny nose stems from a cold or allergies, you'll want to find an effective treatment before your local drugstore runs out of tissues.

Runny Nose Treatment Alternatives: Side-by-Side Comparison

	Conventional Remedy	Treatment Alternative
Generic Treatment	Pseudoephedrine and chlorpheniramine maleate	*Allium cepa*
Sample Brand Name Treatment	Children's Triaminic Cold & Allergy syrup	Children's Coldcalm pellets (Boiron)
How it works	Contains antihistamine and nasal decongestant to relieve runny nose	Temporarily relieves runny nose symptoms
Dosage	Under 4: do not take unless directed by a doctor; age 6-12: 2 tsp every four hours	Under 3: Ask a doctor (typically three pellets 3 times per day); over 3: five pellets every 20 minutes for one hour, then five pellets every two hours until symptoms relieved

	Conventional Remedy	Treatment Alternative
Active Ingredients	Phenylephrine and Chlorpheniramine Maleate	*Allium cepa* 3C, apis mellifica 6C, belladonna 6C, *Eupatorium perfoliatum* 3C, *Gelsemium sempervirens* 6C, kali bichromicum 6C, *nux vomica* 3C, *Phytolacca decandra* 6C, *Pulsatilla* 6C
Common Mild Side Effects	Nervousness, dizziness, sleeplessness	None
Less Common Serious Side Effects	Ears ringing, blurry vision, memory problems	None

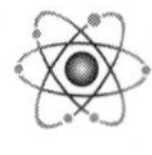

Science Says

Researchers in India conducted a case-series study of the homeopathic treatment of recurrent upper respiratory tract infections (URTIs) in children below the age of 5. They found a statistically significant reduction in the number of attacks of URTIs in the six months preceding and following the date of commencement of homeopathic treatment.

Natural Selection

Home remedies abound for tackling a runny nose. The most helpful suggestions are …

- Nettle tea—boil water and drop in some nettle herb to ease nasal passage inflammation, congestion, and itchiness.

- Saline solution—dissolve ½ teaspoon of non-iodized (sea) salt into a 4-ounce glass of warm distilled water. Use a nose dropper to insert a few drops into each nostril. A neti pot, a small teapot-shaped device that holds the salt water, can be used in children as young as 3 years old to assist in flushing out nasal passages. The neti pot is also a handy tool for treating stuffy noses and sinusitis, conditions covered later in this chapter.
- Thyme—crush a tablespoon of thyme as finely as possible, then gently inhale the powdered thyme.

Sinusitis (Sinus Infection)

Has your kid ever complained of facial pressure? This is not to be confused with peer pressure. Severe pressure in and around the nose and eyes may be a telltale symptom of sinusitis, an inflammation of the nasal passages or sinuses.

Most often caused by a viral infection, sinusitis may also be triggered by pollutants or allergens. For those suffering from severe acute or chronic sinusitis, bacteria or fungi may also be present.

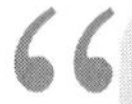

Parental Guidance

"One of the best remedies for us during the cold season or if any of us get a sinus-type infection is drinking a combination of hot water (or herbal tea) mixed with the juice of a fresh squeezed organic lemon, a heaping tablespoon of local raw honey, and a tablespoon (or as much as you can stand) of raw apple cider vinegar at least three times a day. In about three days we are much better, if not completely well again!"
—Kimberly, mom to 5-year-old daughter and 2-year-old son

Beyond facial pressure, your child may also experience headache, stuffy nose, sore throat, cough, or fever when battling sinusitis. Nasal drainage may be all sorts of Day-Glo colors, like fluorescent green and yellow. Let's look at the conventional treatments and alternatives to relieve that pressure.

Sinusitis Treatment Alternatives: Side-by-Side Comparison

	Conventional Remedy	Treatment Alternative
Generic Treatment	Amoxicillin, clavulinic acid	Andrographis extract
Sample Brand Name Treatment	Augmentin	HerbPharm Andrographis
How it works	Helps treat the existing bacterial infection by destroying the outer walls of bacteria cells	Helps boost the immune system's response to infections such as sinusitis
Dosage	Under 88 lbs: consult a doctor for dosage; over 88 lbs: 500mg every 12 hours or 250mg every 8 hours (dosage may also vary by severity of infection)	Add 30-40 drops into water and drink 2-4 times per day.
Active Ingredients	Amoxicillin, clavulanate potassium	*Andrographis paniculata* extractives
Common Mild Side Effects	Rash, diarrhea, unsettled stomach, vomiting	None
Less Common Serious Side Effects	Allergic reaction, yeast infection, difficulty breathing, severe rash	None

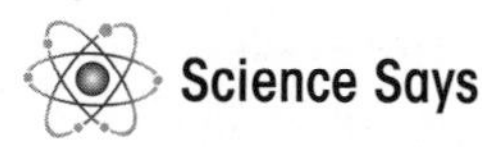

Researchers at the Erubini Medical Center in Armenia conducted a double-blind, placebo-controlled study of Andrographis extracts in the treatment of acute upper respiratory tract infections including sinusitis. Ninety individuals were treated over five days with a placebo or the herb, and final analysis showed significant improvements in the medicated group versus controls including reduced symptoms of headache and nasal/throat symptoms.

Natural Selection

If Andrographis extract isn't your cup of tea, you can also consider one of these three treatment alternatives:

- Mix two tablespoons of organic apple cider vinegar with water and drink to alleviate sinus pressure and congestion.
- Mix two to three drops of grapefruit seed extract with water and drink to promote healing of the infection and symptom relief.
- Increase consumption of ginger, mustard, onions, and horseradish, as these foods are known to help break down mucus.

Stuffy Nose

Earlier in this chapter we covered the runny nose. Let's now delve into the opposite: a stuffy nose. Equally unpleasant to its opposite cousin, the stuffy nose is one of the most prevalent common cold ailments.

A stuffy nose is typically caused by one of many different viruses or allergens. Some may be airborne, but most frequently transmission occurs through hand-to-nose contact. Once your nose absorbs the virus or allergen, the body releases histamine, a chemical that causes nasal tissue to swell. The swelling in turn inflames the nasal membranes, causing excessive mucus to build up and stuff up your nose.

Parental Guidance

"We use eucalyptus and thyme essential oils in a humidifier to ease congestion and cold symptoms, or you can go ahead and put the essential oils in a boiling pot of water and allow the child to breathe the oils in (of course, supervised)."

—Kristina, mother to Mariah, age 12, and Nicolas, age 19 months, and founder of Poofy Organics (www.poofyorganics.com)

When your child loses one of two main air passages for breathing, immediate treatment catapults to the top of your list. That said, let's check out conventional versus natural treatment options.

Stuffy Nose Treatment Alternatives: Side-by-Side Comparison

	Conventional Remedy	Treatment Alternative
Generic Treatment	Pseudoephedrine	Saline drops/spray
Sample Brand Name Treatment	Children's Sudafed Nasal Decongestant	Little Noses Saline Spray/Drops
How it works	Temporarily relieves nasal congestion	Helps loosen and thin mucus secretions
Dosage	Under 4: do not use; 4-5 years: 1 tsp every 4 to 6 hours; 6-11 years: 2 tsp every 4 to 6 hours	Newborns/infants: 2-6 drops per nostril; children: 2-6 sprays per nostril
Active Ingredients	Pseudoephedrine	Sodium chloride
Common Mild Side Effects	Nervousness, dizziness, sleeplessness	Mild irritation

	Conventional Remedy	Treatment Alternative
Less Common Serious Side Effects	Allergic reaction such as hives, difficulty breathing, swelling of the mouth	None

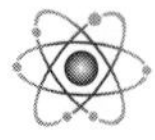

Science Says

The Department of Pediatrics at Chung Shan Medical University Hospital in Taiwan studied the effectiveness of saline in treating rhinosinusitis in children. Of 69 children observed, the half that received saline treatment (versus a placebo control) showed significantly greater resolution of rhinorrhea, nasal congestion, throat itching, cough, and sleep quality.

Natural Selection

If you're looking beyond saline spray and drops for a natural stuffy nose treatment plan, here are three additional home remedies to clear that pesky nasal passage:

- Steam shower—fog up the mirror and let the steam circulate in and around the nasal passage for several minutes.
- Cardiovascular exercise—instead of resting through a stuffy nose, hit the treadmill (or the playground) to stimulate better circulation to purge mucus.
- Spicy foods—some folks believe spicy, peppery, and pungent foods act as natural decongestants.

Swimmer's Ear

If only swimmer's ear referred to the talent of exceptional hearing underwater, childhood games of underwater operator would be popular across the land.

Unfortunately, swimmer's ear (also called otitis externa) is actually a painful infection of the ear canal. It typically occurs when bacteria develops when the thin lining inside the ear canal breaks. This break is usually the result of moisture trapped in the ear canal or an ear trauma such as a deep scratch.

If your child feels pain when the affected ear is touched or when he chews, this may be an indicator of swimmer's ear. Other possible symptoms include ear redness, itching, drainage, clogging, or even difficulty hearing. If your child has been diagnosed with swimmer's ear, consider these conventional and natural treatment options.

Swimmer's Ear Treatment Alternatives: Side-by-Side Comparison

	Conventional Remedy	Treatment Alternative
Generic Treatment	Ciproflaxacin and dexamethasone otic	Acetic acid
Sample Brand Name Treatment	Ciprodex	Spectrum Naturals Organic Apple Cider Vinegar
How it works	Contains an antibiotic to kill bacteria and a steroid to reduce inflammation in the ear canal	The vinegar has anti-inflammatory and anti-bacterial properties.
Dosage	Under 6 months: do not use without consulting a doctor; over 6 months 4 drops (0.14mL) into the: affected ear 2 times per day for 7 days	Put a few drops of vinegar into the affected ear while child lays down with ear facing upward.

	Conventional Remedy	Treatment Alternative
Active Ingredients	Ciprofloxacin, dexamethasone	Organic raw unpasteurized filtered apple cider vinegar
Common Mild Side Effects	Slight itching, taste perversion, discomfort of the ear	None
Less Common Serious Side Effects	Rash, decreased hearing, worsening pain, allergic reaction	None

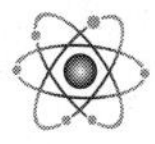

Science Says

Researchers at the Department of Otolaryngology at Stepping Hill Hospital in Stockport, England, assessed the effectiveness of various interventions for acute otitis externa. Acetic acid, the primary ingredient in apple cider vinegar, proved effective and comparable to antibiotic/steroid treatments within the first week of treatment.

Natural Selection

Instead of apple cider vinegar, you can heat a crushed garlic clove in olive oil. Then allow the oil to cool to room temperature, enough to be safe to instill in your child's ear. Strain the garlic pieces and place a few drops of the garlic oil into the painful ear every four hours as needed until the ache is gone. Another simple and effective remedy that can be bought at any drugstore is hydrogen peroxide. Place three or four drops of hydrogen peroxide liquid into the affected ear every four hours as needed for pain.

Spotlight On: Garlic

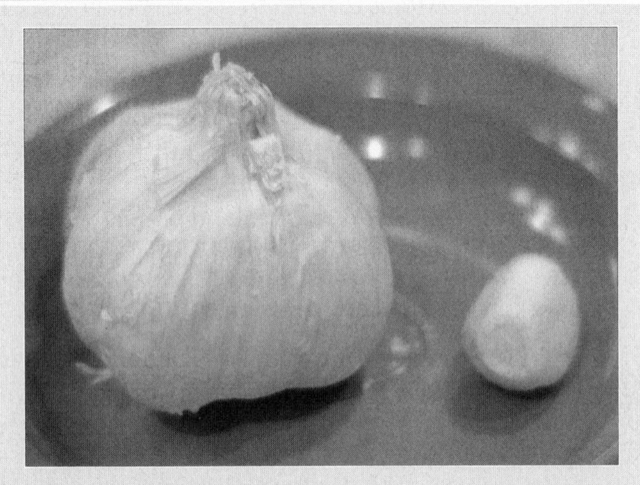

Garlic has many known health benefits.

"Let food be thy medicine and medicine be thy food," is a famous quote from Hippocrates. You may remember this Greek healer not just as the father of Western medicine but also as the man behind the Hippocratic oath. Could one of the most famous historic physicians have had garlic in mind at the time of this quote?

Garlic has been used throughout history to treat many conditions including hypertension, infections, and even snakebites. In fact, some cultures even believed it could ward off unwanted spirits. Halloween aside, garlic has shown positive outcomes in reducing cholesterol levels and cardiovascular risk.

So how does a yummy spice commonly sprinkled on pizza earn praise as a food-based medicinal wonder treatment? Apparently, garlic has a high concentration of sulfur-containing compounds, particularly allicin. It's the allicin that creates the health benefits. In numerous studies over the last 15 to 20 years, allicin has been shown to normalize lipoprotein balance, decrease blood pressure, have anti-inflammatory benefits, and even function as an antioxidant.

Recent studies have also found garlic to be a powerful natural antibiotic. Apparently, the bacteria in the body is less likely to build resistance to garlic than to many lab -developed antibiotics. While the antibiotic benefit is broad-based as opposed to targeted like traditional antibiotics, it's comforting to know the positive health benefits can continue over time.

4

Take Your Breath Away

"The recent increase in allergies and asthma in children comes from environmental causes and triggers—which means there are environmental solutions. Even how kids eat can decrease their risk of asthma and of asthma attacks. For instance, in an Italian study of over 18,000 children, eating fruit rich in vitamin C five to seven times a week was associated with a dramatic reduction in overall wheezing, chronic cough, nighttime cough, and severe wheezing episodes."

—Alan Greene, MD, FAAP, Founder DrGreene.com

We sure do take our breath for granted—except when it's taken away. It's amazing how allergies and coughs can interrupt a seemingly simple daily action like breathing. Suddenly, all your child can think about is wheezing and phlegm.

This chapter is all about ailments that can take your breath away. From allergies and asthma to coughs and pneumonia, the conditions covered in this chapter turn simple breathing into a labored activity.

If your child is coughing right now, you'll want to read this chapter closely to identify the right ailment and best course of treatment. Here's hoping the coughing and wheezing can be replaced with clear breathing and restful nights of sleep.

Allergies (Seasonal)

Ahhhh, springtime! Flowers blooming, green leaves blossoming, temperatures rising. But wait: not everyone cherishes the end of winter. Allergy sufferers would gladly endure another snowstorm if it meant an extra day with clear nasal passages.

Spring and fall most frequently trigger seasonal allergies, an immune system response when the body mistakenly interprets substances like tree, grass, and plant pollens as bodily threats. The body's immune system treats these irritants as it would germs associated with a cold or flu—it releases antibodies and histamines. It's these histamines that generate the allergy symptoms your child experiences.

The most common symptoms include congestion, coughing, runny nose, sneezing, and watery or itchy eyes. These symptoms are most often triggered by pollens and mold. If your child suffers from seasonal allergies, and would prefer living exclusively in summer and winter, then check out these treatment options.

Allergies Treatment Alternatives: Side-by-Side Comparison

	Conventional Remedy	Treatment Alternative
Generic Treatment	Loratidine	Quercetin, stinging nettle, N-acetyl cysteine, bromelain
Sample Brand Name Treatment	Claritin Children's, 24 Hour Allergy, Great Grape	Ortho Molecular D-Hist Jr.
How it works	Contains an antihistamine that helps provide relief from allergy symptoms	Inhibits mast cell degranulation and reduces viscosity of mucus

	Conventional Remedy	Treatment Alternative
Dosage	Children 2 to under 6 years of age: 1 tsp daily; do not take more than 1 tsp in 24 hours; children 6 years and over: 2 tsp daily; do not take more than 2 tsp in 24 hours	Take 1-2 chewable tablets per day or as directed by a doctor.
Active Ingredients	Loratidine	Quercetin, stinging nettle, N-acetyl cysteine, bromelain
Common Mild Side v	Drowsiness, dry mouth, excitability, diarrhea, headache, nausea, vomiting, constipation, decreased appetite	None
Less Common Serious Side Effects	Difficulty urinating, irregular heartbeat, chills, seizure, vision changes, tremor, unexplained bruising or bleeding	Allergic reaction

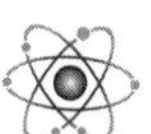

Science Says

Quercetin's effect on allergies is unmatched by other natural substances. It has been shown to prevent the influx of calcium into mast cells and basophils, thereby keeping histamine and other preformed mediators from being released. Stinging nettle leaves block both lipoxygenase and cyclooxygenase, enzymes that increase inflammatory prostaglandins and leukotrienes. N-acetyl L-cysteine (NAC) is an extraordinary antioxidant and mucoregulator.

Natural Selection

If seasonal allergies persist, your child can always try one of these additional treatment alternatives:

- Use a neti pot with non-iodized salt in distilled warm water to flush out the nasal passages and alleviate congestion.
- Eat small daily doses of locally produced honey (for those children one year and older). Honey produced by bees theoretically contains bits of local flower pollens that can act to desensitize sensitive immune systems and help your child more easily tolerate seasonal pollen exposures.
- Increase consumption of foods rich in omega-3 fatty acids, such as salmon, flaxseeds, or walnuts (assuming your child is not allergic to these foods), known for anti-inflammatory actions.

Asthma

Here's a quick test. Can you name the most common chronic condition that affects children? Here's a hint: the answer has something to do with the section you're reading right now. You guessed it. Asthma is the most common chronic condition and typically shows up around the age of five. According to the Centers for Disease Control (CDC), U.S. children miss nearly 13 million days of school per year due to asthma complications.

Asthma affects your child's ability to breath due to inflammation and subsequent narrowing of the airways. The most common symptoms include wheezing, difficulty breathing, or tightness in the chest. An asthma attack occurs when the wheezing is severe, coughing is uncontrollable, or your child experiences paleness, sweating, chest pain, rapid breathing, or an inability to catch his breath.

Some researchers believe there is a link between asthma and genetics, certain foods, obesity, or even environmental factors such as air pollution, allergies, tobacco exposure, and stress. However your child develops asthma, the most important goal is prevention, followed closely by successful acute and chronic management. Here are the conventional and alternative treatment options.

Asthma Treatment Alternatives: Side-by-Side Comparison

	Conventional Remedy	Treatment Alternative
Generic Treatment	Fluticisone	Chinese licorice root and other traditional Chinese medicine (TCM) herbals
Sample Brand Name Treatment	Flovent MDI	Kan Herbals Deep Breath
How it works	Inhalation decreases inflammation and hyperactivity of the airways while decreasing mucus production.	Strengthens lung function and helps reduce wheezing and excessive phlegm
Dosage	Under 4 years: consult a doctor; Over 4 years: 88mcg up to 2 times per day	0-4 years: 15-30 drops, 4-8 years: 30-45 drops, 8-12 years: 45-60 drops, 12+ years: 60-90 drops, 2-3 times per day
Active Ingredients	Fluticasone propionate	Licorice root, cynanchum root and rhizome, platycodon root, purple aster root, stemona root, linula flower, schisandra fruit, mume fruit, white mulberry leaf, white mulberry bark, peucedanum root, dried ginger rhizome, Chinese licorice root, treated Pinellia rhizome, dong quai root, dried rind of mature tangerine fruit, white Asian ginseng root

	Conventional Remedy	Treatment Alternative
Common Mild Side Effects	Throat irritation, upper respiratory tract infection, headache, bronchitis, thrush, vomiting, fever, nausea, cough, weight gain, high blood sugar, depression	None
Less Common Serious Side Effects	Stunted growth, urinary tract infection, muscle or bone pain, migraine, digestive pain, blurred vision, numbness, allergic reaction	Allergic reaction

Science Says

Researchers in the Department of Pediatrics at Mount Sinai School of Medicine in New York reviewed five clinical studies of anti-asthma TCM herbal remedies, including licorice root extracts. Speculated mechanisms for activity include anti-inflammation, inhibition of airway smooth muscle contraction, and immunomodulation. The NIH's National Center for Complementary and Alternative Medicine (NCCAM) published a statement on the use of traditional Chinese medicine (TCM) herbals for asthma treatment, noting, "Preliminary clinical trials of formulas containing *Radix glycyrrhizae* (licorice root) in combination with various other TCM herbs have had positive results. All of the trials reported improvement in lung function with the herbal formulas and found them to be safe and well tolerated."

Natural Selection

John D. Mark, MD, Clinical Professor of Pediatrics (Division of Pulmonary Medicine) at Stanford University School of Medicine, notes, "By using mind-body therapies such as relaxation and guided imagery, I have found that many children and young adults with asthma have been able to decrease their use of rescue medications. Many of these same patients have also been able to lower the dose or even discontinue controller medications such as inhaled corticosteroids."

Looking for additional natural alternatives for your child's asthma symptoms? Make sure she's getting plenty of vitamin D—research has clearly demonstrated that children with low vitamin D levels are more likely to suffer from asthma. Also, increase intake of fruits and vegetables—rich in natural antioxidant vitamins and minerals—to help prevent and reduce asthma exacerbations.

Bronchitis

Anytime your kid starts coughing, you immediately wonder if it's bronchitis. That ailment must have done some seriously impressive marketing to be so top of mind among parents.

Truth be told, not every cough equals bronchitis. Defined as an inflammation of the bronchial tubes, bronchitis occurs when the airways and trachea become inflamed from infection or irritation, thereby affecting the way air is carried to and from the lungs.

There are two types of bronchitis: acute and chronic. Acute bronchitis usually occurs during the course of a viral illness such as the common cold or influenza. Chronic bronchitis is characterized by a productive cough that lasts three months or more. It usually develops from a recurrent injury to the airways from an inhaled irritant like smoke or dust or in children with underlying respiratory issues.

Most parents automatically assume bronchitis needs to be treated with antibiotics. In fact, many types of bronchitis are not caused by bacteria but by viruses or allergens and are therefore not treatable with antibiotic therapy.

However your child develops bronchitis, you'll want to know the conventional and alternative treatment options available.

Bronchitis Treatment Alternatives: Side-by-Side Comparison

	Conventional Remedy	Treatment Alternative
Generic Treatment	Azithromycin	Pelargonium
Sample Brand Name Treatment	Zithromax Children's Syrup	Umcka Cold Care
How it works	The antibiotic fights the bacteria associated with bronchitis to fight infection.	Boosts the body's immune system and supports its natural defense system
Dosage	Take one tablet per day for five days with or without food.	Under 2 years: consult a doctor; 2-5 years: ½ tsp 3 times per day; 6-11 years: 1 tsp 3 times per day; over 12 years: 1½ tsp 3 times per day
Active Ingredients	Azithromycin	*Pelargonium sidoides*
Common Mild Side Effects	Upset stomach, diarrhea, vomiting, stomach pain, mild rash	None
Less Common Serious Side Effects	Severe allergic reaction, blurred vision, hearing loss, face swelling, skin yellowing, irregular heartbeat	None

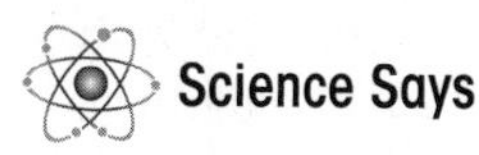

Science Says

Pelargonium is a genus of flowering plants commonly known as scented geraniums or storksbills. The Department of Pneumology at University Hospital in Freiburg, Germany, studied the effectiveness of *Pelargonium sidoides* in the treatment of acute bronchitis using a multi-center, prospective, open observational study design. Over 2,000 patients were given a *Pelargonium sidoides* treatment solution in age-specific dosages for 14 days. Researchers found significantly improved Bronchitis Severity Score (BSS) after treatment. Furthermore, mild adverse events were only reported in 1.2 percent of patients and serious adverse events were reported in none.

Natural Selection

If that coughing just won't quit, you can always get the humidifier from your closet and run it all night long for your child. Diffusing peppermint oil or eucalyptus oil may help ease discomfort as well. During the day, drinking tea with honey, cinnamon, cloves, or ginger can help ease coughing symptoms. If your child can gargle, consider warm salt water to help relieve inflammation and irritation.

Dry Cough

Toddlers and dry coughs go together like orange juice and minty toothpaste. There's nothing like a persistent cough to destroy nighttime sleep, irritate the most mild-mannered youngster, and ultimately challenge the patience of a loving parent.

Rest assured you're not destined to night after night of 3 A.M. wake-ups. Treatments abound to loosen phlegm and alleviate both chest and throat congestion.

Dry and wet cough symptoms and treatment options are not the same, so we'll cover them separately in the next two sections. Dry coughing symptoms are hard to miss. Your child will feel that incessant tickling sensation in his throat. Intense bouts of hacking coughs are common, as are difficulty breathing and even talking.

Parental Guidance

"The staples in my home are Chestal for cough and congestion, elderberry for the common cold, and garlic/olive oil for earaches."

—Allison, mother to 4-year-old boy and 16-month-old girl

Unlike many other ailments covered in this book, a dry cough cannot be traced to one universal cause. Instead, it can be the result of many ailments including the common cold, laryngitis, asthma, bronchitis, upper respiratory tract infections, sinus problems, and even pneumonia.

Regardless of cause, a dry cough that interferes with sleep is better off addressed than ignored. Here are the conventional remedies versus natural equivalents to help your offspring regain a spring in their step.

Dry Cough Treatment Alternatives: Side-by-Side Comparison

	Conventional Remedy	Treatment Alternative
Generic Treatment	Guaifenesin	Homeopathics and honey
Sample Brand Name Treatment	Children's Robitussin Cough	Children's Chestal from Boiron
How it works	An expectorant that loosens congestion in chest and throat	Helps loosen phlegm and thin bronchial secretion to make coughs more productive

	Conventional Remedy	Treatment Alternative
Dosage	Under 4: do not take; 4-6 years: 1 tsp every 6-8 hours; 6-12 years: 2 tsp every 6-8 hours over 12 years: 4 tsp every 6-8 hours	Under 1: not recommended 1-2 years: consult your doctor; 2-12 years: 1 tsp every 2 hours; over 12 years:
Active Ingredients	Guaifenesin, Dextromethorphan	Antimonium tartaricum 6C, *Bryonia alba* 3C, *Coccus cacti* 3C, *Drosera rotundifolia* 3C, *Ipecacuanha* 3C, *Pulsatilla* 6C, *Rumex crispus* 6C, Spongia tosta 3C, *Sticta pulmonaria* 3C
Common Mild Side Effects	Dizziness, headache, rash, nausea, vomiting, upset stomach	None
Less Common Serious Side Effects	Allergic reaction	Allergic reaction to honey

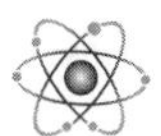

Science Says

Researchers in Austria compared the safety and efficacy of homeopathic treatments for cough and acute respiratory complaints in children and adults. The onset of improvement within the first seven days after treatment was significantly faster with homeopathic versus conventional treatment. Also, the Department of Pediatrics at the Shahid Sadoughi University of Medical Sciences in Iran conducted a comparison of the effect of honey, dextromethorphan, and diphenhydramine on nightly cough and sleep quality in children and their parents. After studying 139 children, ages 24 to 60 months, researchers found honey to be more effective in controlling cough symptoms compared to conventional treatments. Additionally, honey-treated children slept more soundly.

Natural Selection

Maty's All Natural Baby Chest Rub is another great option for alleviating dry cough symptoms. It contains a proprietary blend of essential oils, including eucalyptus, lavender, and chamomile, to boost immune function while calming cough symptoms. Your child can also drink a combination of decaffeinated green tea and honey to decrease coughing spells. Finally, a mixture of turmeric with warm water or milk can help your child sleep more restfully and ease a cough.

Wet Cough

"Mommy, I thought mucus is supposed to be in my nose!" You assure her that's its usual home. "Then why do I feel it in my mouth when I cough?" Your seven-year-old just scored a quick education in the wet cough. Defined by that phlegmy feeling in your chest, wet coughs are the opposite of dry but are equally uncomfortable for your little one.

Wet coughs result from the presence of excess mucus in the upper or lower respiratory tract. It can impact the lungs, bronchi, larynx, or pharynx. Wet coughs often tag along with other common ailments such as a cold, the flu, or even hay fever.

✓ Good to Know

Phlegm is the key differentiator between a dry and wet cough. No phlegm equals dry, loads of phlegm equals wet. It's nice to know such a simple distinction can point you toward the right treatment. You'll never look at phlegm the same!

Since wet coughs have the distinct symptom of that phlegmy feeling in your throat and chest, let's dig deeper into the causes. The most common include the following:

- An infection in your child's upper airway passage or lungs
- A viral illness (e.g., the common cold) that leads to mucus draining down your child's throat
- Postnasal drip seeping down the back of your child's throat
- Stomach acid backing up (refluxing) in the esophagus, causing excess mucus production in the throat and upper airway

We've got the symptoms and causes clear for wet coughs; let's now look more closely at treatment options.

Wet Cough Treatment Alternatives: Side-by-Side Comparison

	Conventional Remedy	Treatment Alternative
Generic Treatment	Brompheniramine maleate, Dextromethorphan HBr, Phenylephrine HCl	Chamomile tea
Sample Brand Name Treatment	Children's Dimetapp Cold & Cough	Traditional Medicinals Organic Chamomile Tea
How it works	Temporarily relieves cough due to minor throat and bronchial irritation occurring with a cold, and nasal congestion	Soothes sore throat associated with persistent cough
Dosage	Under 6: Do not use; 6-12 years: 2 tsp every 4 hrs; over 12 years: 4 tsp every 4 hrs	1-2 cups per day as needed
Active Ingredients	Brompheniramine maleate, Dextromethorphan HBr, Phenylephrine HCl	Chamomile

	Conventional Remedy	Treatment Alternative
Common Mild Side Effects	Drowsiness, dizziness, headache, restlessness	None
Less Common Serious Side Effects	Blurred vision, tremor, trouble urinating	None

Science Says

The Department of Pharmacology at Helwan University in Egypt studied the effect of an herbal-water extract (including chamomile, saffron, anise, fennel, caraway, licorice, cardamom, and black seed) on cough. The herbal mixture, compared to a placebo tea, led to significant improvements in cough frequency and intensity as well as a reduction in sleep discomfort.

Natural Selection

Think hot, hot, hot when it comes to home remedies for breaking up a nasty wet cough. Grandma's chicken noodle soup, hot water or tea, and lounging in a steam shower all help break up signature wet cough phlegm. It turns out that chicken soup actually works to decrease the inflammatory response (thereby reducing phlegm production) by inhibiting neutrophils (a type of white blood cell) migration, according to one study by researchers from the Pulmonary and Critical Care Medicine Section at the Nebraska Medical Center.

Croup

"Daddy, why is Eddie barking like a seal?" Little sisters do have a way with words. "He's got a case of croup, honey; he can't help it."

Croup causes inflammation in the upper airways, notably the vocal chords and windpipe. That barking cough or hoarseness is the signature sign for croup.

Croup is typically caused by a virus and is both most common and most severe in children 6 months to 3 years of age. Older kids can also catch croup, though it's less common.

It's possible to at first confuse croup with the common cold. It often begins with cold-like symptoms such as stuffy nose and fever. However, soon enough that seal-like barking begins—usually in the wee hours of the morning, of course—and you know it's time to choose a croup treatment plan.

Croup Treatment Alternatives: Side-by-Side Comparison

	Conventional Remedy	Treatment Alternative
Generic Treatment	Prednisone	Eucalyptus Oil
Sample Brand Name Treatment	Orapred	Young Living Eucalyptus Oil
How it works	Helps reduce upper airway swelling	Helps thin mucus in the lungs and airway
Dosage	1-2 mg/kg per day	A few drops diluted into vaporizer or steam
Active Ingredients	Prednisone, alcohol	Eucalyptus leaves
Common Mild Side Effects	Dizziness, headache, acne, heartburn, insomnia, sweating	Asthma-like symptoms
Less Common Serious Side Effects	Extreme mood changes, bulging eyes, skin blotches, irregular menstrual cycles	None

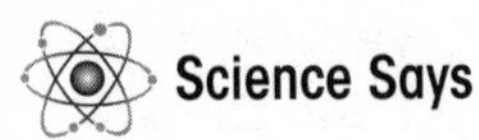

Science Says

According to Natural Medicines Comprehensive Database, eucalyptus oil appears to have both analgesic and anti-inflammatory effects without the more dangerous side effects associated with conventional treatments like prednisone. One published study, from the Department of Family Medicine at the Technion-Israel Institute of Technology in Haifa, Israel, demonstrated rapid cough and hoarseness symptom relief with treatment from an essential-oil-based spray primarily containing eucalyptus.

Natural Selection

If eucalyptus oil doesn't do the job, consider a homeopathic remedy called aconitum. Derived from the flowering plant in the buttercup family commonly known as monkshood or wolfsbane, homeopathic aconitum is available in several dilutions in pellet form; the 30c dilution is often used acutely for croup. Aconitum is classically used by homeopaths to treat conditions marked by a state of fear and anxiety with "anguish of mind and body." In fact, many children with croup do appear anxious and fearful, as do their parents.

Pneumonia

"Put your jacket on—it's 40 degrees outside! Do you want to catch pneumonia?" Parents sure do know how to warn their kids about the risk of pneumonia.

Of course, there's more to it than the jacket decision. Pneumonia refers to inflammation or an infection in one or both lungs and can be caused by a number of factors including viruses, bacteria, or even foreign matter (food or fluid) that reaches the lungs after aspiration.

The most common form of pneumonia in children is viral pneumonia, which typically stems from the flu. Your child may experience a host of symptoms including cough, high fever, congestion, chest or abdominal pain, vomiting, labored breathing, listlessness, lack of appetite, diarrhea, fussiness, or pale blue coloring of the lips and fingernails.

Parental Guidance

"When Phoenix starts to get a cold we immediately start taking oregano oil. I rub it on the bottom of his feet and my husband and I take it internally in a capsule. Oregano is so powerful and helps our bodies fight whatever germs are mustering up strength. I also spend the next few nights cooking with a lot of extra garlic. We will eat garlic hummus, pasta sauces, and use it in omelets. Because garlic helps strengthen our immune systems I know that we are fueling our bodies with something healthy. If I start early enough this combination almost always prevents a major illness."

—Lauren, mom to 15 month old boy

With this laundry list of symptoms, you'll want to battle back against pneumonia right away to help your child feel better. Here are some of the treatment options available. Note that antibiotics are essential in the treatment of bacterial pneumonia. In that case, we recommend the natural remedies listed here be used as complements, not alternatives, to conventional treatment. This is true integrative medicine in action. It's also important to clarify that pneumonia, just like sinus and ear infections, can be viral or bacterial. Viral infections do not need to be—and should not be—treated with antibiotics.

Pneumonia Treatment Alternatives: Side-by-Side Comparison

	Conventional Remedy	Treatment Alternative
Generic Treatment	Cefuroxime	Zinc Sulfate
Sample Brand Name Treatment	Ceftin (liquid) sulfate	Thorne Research Zinc Sulfate
How it works	Stops the production of bacteria associated with pneumonia (not prescribed for viral pneumonia)	Provides zinc to support immune function
Dosage	Ages 3 months to 12 years: take twice per day for 10 days in the amount prescribed by a medical professional based on age, weight, and type of infection	Ages 0-3 years: 5-10mg zinc intake per day; ages 4-10 years: 10mg zinc intake per day; over 11 years: 12-15mg zinc intake per day
Active Ingredients	Cefuroxime axetil	Zinc sulfate
Common Mild Side Effects	Vomiting, diarrhea, upset stomach	Nausea, headache, upset stomach, heartburn
Less Common Serious Side Effects	Severe vomiting or diarrhea, allergic reaction, yeast infection, sores in mouth or throat, unusual bleeding, seizure	Toxicity due to zinc overdose

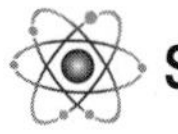

Science Says

Researchers in the Department of Pediatrics at the Jundishapour University of Medical Sciences in Iran studied the efficacy of zinc sulfate supplementation on the outcome of children with severe pneumonia. In the study, 128 children ages 3 to 60 months old were divided into two groups. One received zinc sulfate for five days, the other received a placebo. The zinc treated group experienced significantly shorter duration of fever and respiratory distress as well as shorter hospital stays. Additionally, the zinc supplement was well tolerated.

Natural Selection

If zinc isn't your cup of tea, consider adding Schisandra berries, from the magnolia vine, to any herbal infusion. These berries have long been used in traditional Chinese medicine as a lung tonic.

Vitamin and mineral deficiencies contribute to weakened immune systems, leaving children vulnerable to severe bacterial infections. For example, kids with vitamin D deficiency seem to suffer more severe lower respiratory tract infections. Extra vitamin D_3 during the winter may help reduce your child's risk of pneumonia. One study in Bangladesh demonstrated that children hospitalized with pneumonia provided micronutrients (vitamin A, vitamin C, vitamin E, folic acid, and zinc) fared better than controls.

Spotlight On: Honey

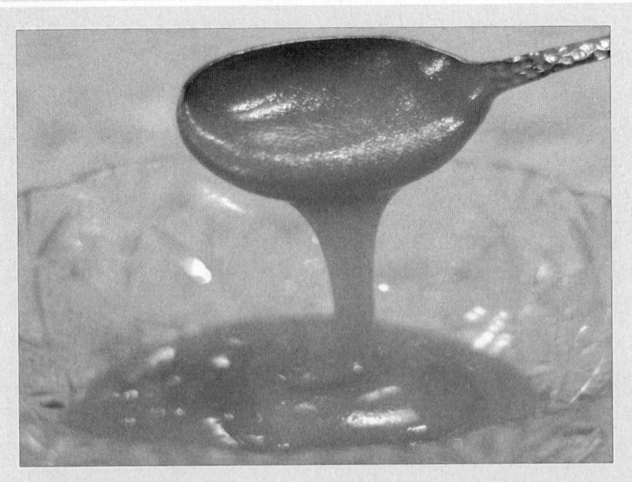

Honey can be used as a safe cough and cold treatment.

Winnie-the-Pooh had it all figured out—it's all about the honey. People over many centuries have gathered this tasty, sticky delight to treat everything from coughs and sniffles to sneezes and runny noses. Honey may, in fact, be nature's safest over-the-counter cough and cold treatment and its most potent antibiotic—all without the potentially dangerous side effects of conventional medications.

Coughing is the body's way of clearing irritated airways to help your child breathe more comfortably. However, persistent coughing may only irritate the lungs and throat further. All that hacking prevents a restful night's sleep, something parents everywhere want for their little ones.

With all that coughing, it's no wonder parents reach for whatever can ease the symptoms. However, the American Academy of Pediatrics has warned that codeine and dextromethorphan, two common cough medicine ingredients, offer little help for young children. Complications such as drowsiness, headaches, and hyperactivity are common, and more serious adverse effects, like respiratory depression, can happen with overdosing.

Enter honey. You likely think of it as a tasty subsitute for sugar in coffee and tea. Turns out its healing powers may come from the sticky consistency that helps coat and soothe the throat. It may also be the honey's antioxidants that protect our cells from damage. Studies have shown that antioxidant levels rise after honey consumption. The darker honeys, such as buckwheat honey, contain the highest antioxidant concentrations. More recently, research has proven specific honeys (like New Zealand Manuka) to have powerful antibacterial properties that assist in wound healing.

So while there's no evidence that honey has cold prevention benefits, it sure seems worth a try the next time your little one starts hacking or needs a topical wound antiseptic.

5

Temperature Rising

"I tell parents all the time not to fear a fever. Fever itself is not the disease, it is a normal, healthy response. Fevers are such a wonderful way for the body to burn off infection, cleanse the body and naturally boost your immune system. Most fevers can be managed with plenty of fluids, tepid sponge baths, botanical medicines and essential oils."

—Pina LoGiudice ND, LAc, Co-medical director, Inner Source Natural Health, NYC (www.InnerSourceHealth.com)

"Quick! Run to the medicine cabinet and grab the thermometer." What loving parent hasn't uttered these words when confronted with a feverish child? Sure, a kiss to the forehead is the unscientific method for temperature calculation; however, in the digital age, we want accurate documentation to the decimal point. After all, 100.3 and 103.5 aren't just competing radio stations; to us, they're drastically different temperatures requiring specific treatment protocol. To most doctors, a fever is no reason to panic, but we all want children to be comfortable.

This chapter is all about fever, flu, and mononucleosis, three ailments that bring the thermometer into play. For each, we'll be reviewing the conventional remedies and treatment alternatives to nurse your child back to health.

If you're looking for something more than the forehead-kiss diagnosis plan, this is the chapter for you.

Fever

Fever in children is categorized as a temperature of 100° Fahrenheit or higher (when temperature is taken orally). Temperature can be determined orally, rectally, or under the armpit. Some thermometers even capture temperature across the forehead via the temporal artery.

Parental Guidance

"The week my daughter turned 1 year old, she developed a terrible cold and high fever. When her fever got especially high, I took her into a steamy bathroom and applied peppermint essential oil on the soles of her feet. Within minutes, her fever broke and she fell asleep peacefully in my arms. I spent the rest of the week carrying her in a sling and nursing her."

—Erica, mother to Leo and Ilana and founder of "Nature Girl Wellness"

Parental Guidance

"Whenever my baby or children have high fever and I want the temperature to drop, I coat the bottom of their feet with olive oil (cover liberally as garlic can burn through skin) and put some crushed garlic paste and wrap their feet in plastic wrap to hold the garlic paste in place. I leave it on for a couple of hours (preferably during sleep so not to move feet). It's potent and very effective."

—Melody, mother of four boys, Gabriel, Mason, Ryker, and Asher

Fever is often a symptom of a minor health ailment like a viral infection. The main symptom of a fever is a child being warm to the touch, specifically on the cheeks or forehead. Other symptoms may include sweating; headache; exhaustion; changes in eating, drinking, or breathing; chills; fussiness; crying; and aches and pains. It's important to know that fever itself is rarely dangerous—it's usually a sign that the body is fighting against infection. The major reason to treat fever, if need be, is to keep your child comfortable.

Parental Guidance

"When he was younger, my now 2-year-old had very frequent high fevers that seemed to only be able to get under control with ibuprofen. I never felt comfortable giving him a medication with so many possible side effects, but the fevers made him suffer and we couldn't just wait it out (believe me, I always waited until the last moment hoping the fever would come down on its own or with everything else we tried—including cold wash cloths, essential oils, belladonna, etc.). I finally tried *Aconitum napellus* and the fever went down gently."

—Petra, mom to 2-year-old Thies and 5-year-old Ian

Now that we know the causes of and symptoms associated with fever, let's look into the conventional remedies and treatment alternatives to get your kid back to 98.6°.

Fever Side-by-Side Comparison

	Conventional Remedy	Treatment Alternative
Generic Treatment	Acetaminophen	Water
Sample Brand Name Treatment	Children's Tylenol	N/A
How it works	Tylenol contains ingredients that reduce pain and fever in children ages 2-11.	Water helps rid the body of toxins while also preventing dehydration.

	Conventional Remedy	Treatment Alternative
Dosage	See package for dosage instructions; under 2 years: consult a doctor; 2-3 years: 1 tsp; 4-5 years 1.5 tsp; 6-8 years 2 tsp; 9-10 years: 2.5 tsp; 11 years: 3 tsp; every 4 hours for all. Children over age 2, do not exceed 5 doses in 24 hours.	At least 8 glasses per day as fever persists
Active Ingredients	Acetaminophen	H_2O
Common Mild Side Effects	Constipation, diarrhea, drowsiness, dizziness, headache, nausea, anxiety, weakness, decreased appetite, vomiting	None
Less Common Serious Side Effects	Allergic reaction, dark urine, severe headache or dizziness, tremor, vision impairments, or yellowing skin or eyes	None

Natural Selection

Several homeopathic medicines can be quite effective for fever. Consider Belladonna 30c as another treatment alternative for high fever, especially when associated with pain, flushed skin, and thirst. Simply dissolve three to five pellets under the child's tongue every two to four hours (or as directed by a licensed practitioner). Aconitum is another homeopathic fever remedy, best for fevers associated with acute anxiety or fear. Another natural choice is to drench your child's socks or towels in vinegar or cold water and place around the feet to help bring down a fever. Some naturopaths recommend placing wet socks in the freezer for 30 minutes and then putting them on your child's feet until the socks are no longer cool. Seems a bit drastic but it does the trick.

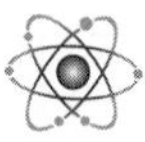

Science Says

According to the American Academy of Pediatrics, "Fever in a child is one of the most common clinical symptoms managed by pediatricians and other health care providers and a frequent cause of parental concern.... [It] is not the primary illness but is a physiologic mechanism that has beneficial effects in fighting infection. There is no evidence that fever itself worsens the course of an illness or that it causes long-term neurologic complications. Thus, the primary goal of treating the febrile child should be to improve the child's overall comfort rather than focus on the normalization of body temperature."

Flu

"Maybe he has a touch of the flu." It's a common concern when your child shows symptoms more severe than the common cold. But how can you tell if that sore throat or malaise is a stand-alone malady or the beginning of the flu? Let's check out the symptoms to get a better sense.

Influenza, more commonly called the flu, is a virus contagious through exposure to an infected person's saliva or other bodily secretions.

Symptoms of the flu may include fever, cough, weakness, sore throat, malaise, body aches, and occasionally vomiting and diarrhea.

Left untreated, the flu may resolve spontaneously or develop into something more serious such as pneumonia.

Parental Guidance

"I have been looking for a natural remedy to ease symptoms of common colds and flu for my two boys. I finally found it in Sambucol (black elderberry extract). It is 10 percent natural, it tastes great, and there are no side effects. And it works! I give it to the kids at the first signs of a cold and two days later, the symptoms disappear!"

—Lana, mother of two boys, ages 3 and 9

While the flu often resolves by itself in time without medication, there are plenty of conventional and natural treatment alternatives. Let's review the most popular.

Flu Side-by-Side Comparison

	Conventional Remedy	Treatment Alternative
Generic Treatment	Oseltamivir	Elderberry
Sample Brand Name Treatment	Tamiflu	Sambucol
How it works	Tamiflu helps treat and prevent the flu by attacking the virus that causes it (for those who have had symptoms less than 2 days).	Sambucol contains antioxidants and other elements that help cure viruses like the flu.
Dosage	See package for dosage instructions; not for children under 1 year of age; less than 34 lbs: 30mg twice per day; 34-51 lbs: 45mg twice per day; 52-88 lbs: 60mg twice per day; 89+ lbs: 75mg twice per day.	Ages 2-3 years: 5mL per day; ages 4-12 years: 10mL per day; do not use on children under 2 years of age.

	Conventional Remedy	Treatment Alternative
Active Ingredients	Oseltamivir phosphate	Black elderberry extract
Common Mild Side Effects	Nausea, vomiting	Nausea
Less Common Serious Side Effects	Allergic reaction, seizures, dark urine, severe headache or dizziness, tremor, vision impairments, or yellowing skin or eyes	None

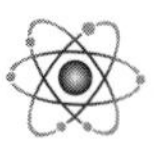

Science Says

The Department of Virology at Hebrew University-Hadassah Medical School in Jerusalem, Israel, conducted a randomized study of the efficacy and safety of oral elderberry extract in the treatment of influenza A and B virus infections. Sixty patients received either 15mL of elderberry or a placebo 4 times per day for five days. Researchers found that symptoms were relieved on average four days earlier for those patients receiving elderberry.

Natural Selection

A child (non-vegetarian) should try consuming chicken broth (made from bones, not the powder substitute) to stay hydrated and to keep something in his or her stomach. Broth may also help loosen mucus. As mentioned in Chapter 4, chicken soup actually contains natural chemicals that help fight infections. Additionally, you can mix thyme and hot water, then let your child sip it to promote a healthy respiratory system and to decrease symptoms such as coughing and sore throat. The most widely used—and hardest to pronounce—homeopathic remedy in the world, oscillococcinum, can lead to relief when given every few hours at the onset of flu-like symptoms.

Mononucleosis

Can you imagine the anticipation your teenager experiences just prior to a first kiss? It's that moment she'll remember forever. We all remember our first kiss—but who could have guessed that a disease would be associated with smooching? Thanks to saliva, something as beautiful as a first kiss is forever linked to mononucleosis.

Mononucleosis, caused by the Epstein-Barr virus, is a contagious virus spread by bodily secretions such as saliva and mucus. It is also referred to as the "kissing disease."

Symptoms of mononucleosis may last weeks or several months. Main symptoms include swollen lymph nodes or tonsils, chills, fever, fatigue, sore throat, liver or spleen inflammation, and decreased appetite.

Mononucleosis is most commonly seen in teenagers and those in their early twenties but is also diagnosed in younger children. While the virus ultimately needs to run its course, medications are generally given to relieve symptoms rather than cure the virus.

Mononucleosis Side-by-Side Comparison

	Conventional Remedy	Treatment Alternative
Generic Treatment	Prednisone	Vitamin C
Sample Brand Name Treatment	Deltasone	Carlson for Kids Chewable Vitamin C
How it works	Deltasone helps decrease symptoms such as swelling and fatigue.	Helps provide support for a healthy immune system
Dosage	Dosage is determined by a doctor; take with food and a full glass of water.	Take 1-4 tablets (250mg each) per day depending on age.
Active Ingredients	Prednisone	Vitamin C (ascorbic acid)

	Conventional Remedy	Treatment Alternative
Common Mild Side Effects	Nausea, vomiting, weakness, weight loss, headache, fatigue, heartburn, dizziness, sweating, acne, insomnia, euphoria	Gastrointestinal distress
Less Common Serious Side Effects	Severe allergic reactions; appetite loss; black, tarry stools; changes in menstrual periods; convulsions; depression; diarrhea; dizziness; exaggerated sense of well-being; fever; general body discomfort; headache; increased pressure in the eye; joint or muscle pain; mood swings; muscle weakness; personality changes; prolonged sore throat, cold, or fever; puffing of the face; severe nausea or vomiting; swelling of feet or legs; unusual weight gain; vomiting material that looks like coffee grounds; weakness; weight loss	None

It should be noted that the incubation period for mono is long, typically 30 to 50 days. In fact, some people who have already had mono can carry the virus in their throats for a while after the illness. They may not even remember being sick anymore, yet they're still contagious.

Ultimately, a mono test (a blood test detecting acute antibodies to Epstein-Barr virus) is the best way to positively confirm the disease. This is an important step since many of the symptoms are shared with other ailments covered in this book. It's important to note that the first mono test can actually be negative but subsequent tests may confirm the disease.

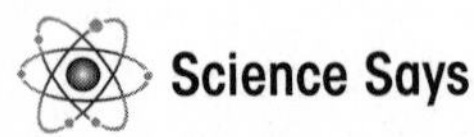

Science Says

The Department of Biotechnology at Kansai University in Osaka, Japan, studied the inhibitory effects of ascorbic acid (vitamin C) on the Epstein-Barr virus (the cause of infectious mononucleosis). Researchers discovered that ascorbic acid exhibited significant effects limiting the activation of the Epstein-Barr virus.

Natural Selection

Children can gargle water mixed with salt to ease a sore throat associated with mononucleosis. Your child can also take the herb milk thistle to promote liver health, which may help an inflamed liver caused by mono. Finally, both vitamin D and probiotics help promote a healthy immune system.

Spotlight On: Hand Sanitizer

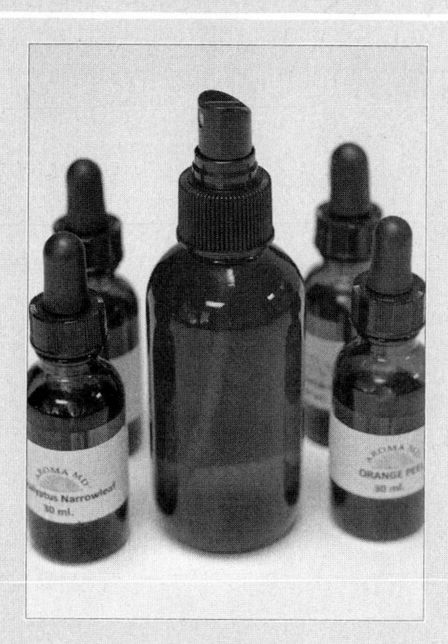

Dr. Rosen's do-it-yourself hand sanitizer.

Hands sure are, well, handy. We use them for eating, picking stuff up, greeting others, and even an impromptu game of patty-cake. It's no wonder one of our most useful body parts is also a germ factory. That's where hand sanitizer comes into play. When rubbed on the hands for 30 seconds, it can kill many forms of bacteria and even some dangerous viruses. Further, hand sanitizer can even retard the redevelopment of bacteria.

Of course, hand sanitizer can't prevent all contact with germs, as many viruses are spread through nasal inhalation. However, the simple hand sanitizer squirt has been linked to decreases in illness rates and improved attendance records at school. Unfortunately, most commerical hand sanitizers contain harsh chemicals like triclosan and alcohol. But nature has provided us with plants and spices with natural antibacterial and antiviral properties.

And that's what led Dr. Rosen to develop his own do-it-yourself hand sanitizer recipe from all-natural ingredients. That's right, this book is not just about ailments, it's also a recipe book! All you need is a 4-ounce spray dispenser filled with 3 ounces of filtered water. Add to it 1 teaspoon of aloe vera gel. Then grab your essential oils and add 10 drops each of cinnamon, clove, rosemary, and eucalyptus oils, plus 20 drops of lemon oil. The result is a natural, chemical-free hand sanitizer to keep germs at bay.

So whether you follow Dr. Rosen's all-natural hand sanitizer recipe, create your own for the kids, or pick something up at the local grocery store, it's clear a few squirts can keep your little squirt healthy.

6

Tummy Troubles

"Mind-body approaches—relaxation, meditation, guided imagery—are fundamental to good digestion and to dealing with "tummy troubles." They go hand-in-hand with the simple, practical dietary changes that Dr. Rosen and Jeff Cohen recommend."

—James S. Gordon, MD, author of *Unstuck: Your Guide to the Seven-Stage Journey Out of Depression,* founder and director of The Center for Mind-Body Medicine, and Dean of the College of Mind-Body Medicine at Saybrook University.

This is a chapter of contrast. Words like *diarrhea* and *constipation* make even the most mild-mannered child giggle. However, when one of these ailments strikes, it's anything but amusing for your little one.

With so many organs and the digestive tract housed in the abdomen, it's no wonder symptoms and treatments can be so confusing. Can your 9-year-old son really pinpoint the difference between nausea and recurrent abdominal pain? It all adds up to, "Mommy, I don't feel too good."

In this chapter, we shall do our best to clarify the multitude of tummy troubles that strike kids. From there we'll describe the causes and symptoms of each, as well as how you can treat the ailments—both conventionally and through treatment alternatives.

So if your son is currently rubbing his tummy and wincing, you'll want to bookmark this chapter. It's your chance to get your kid back to giggling about tummy ailments.

Constipation

Getting your child to sit on the potty is challenging enough; add constipation and you've really got your parental work cut out for you. All pushing with nothing to show for it will frustrate even the most patient child.

Constipation is defined as difficulty in passing stools or the inability to pass stools. Symptoms of constipation include hardened and painful stools, nausea, stomach pain, cramping, or changes in the frequency of urination.

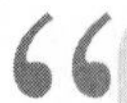

Parental Guidance

"There is a very easy, natural way to relieve constipation with the essential oil, tangerine. We also like to use a Young Living blend called "Di-Gize". Be sure to always use a grade of oil that is food grade (safe enough to ingest). Take a few drops of organic olive oil or other "fatty" oil and apply it to the top of the shin. Rub gently up and down between the knee and the ankle. Keep rubbing the shins; it may take up to 20 minutes to relieve the constipation. Drinking warm water will also help."

—Carrie Donegan & Elena Yordán, authors of the book *Essential Oils 101*.

In children of potty-training age, constipation is common due to avoidance of the toilet. Changes in diet and increased junk food consumption may also cause constipation.

A number of medical conditions may also cause constipation, such as dehydration or cow's milk allergy. Constipation is also a side effect of many medications.

If your child is busy pushing with no results, then you'll definitely want to understand the treatment alternatives available.

Constipation Side-by-Side Comparison

	Conventional Remedy	Treatment Alternative
Generic Treatment	Polyethelene Glycol 3350	Flaxseed Powder
Sample Brand Name Treatment	Miralax	Bob's Red Mill Flaxseed Meal Golden Organic
How it works	Miralax helps soften stools and makes the process of having a bowel movement easier by balancing water in the digestive system.	Flaxseeds work as a natural stool softener.
Dosage	Not intended for children under 2; dose is based on weight and ranges from 2 oz twice daily for children who weigh 22 lbs to 8 oz twice daily for children weighing 110 lbs.	One tbsp daily, best taken with fluids, fruits, or vegetables
Active Ingredients	Polyethelene Glycol 3350	Organic flaxseeds
Common Mild Side Effects	Nausea, cramping, stomach pains, gas, bloating	Gas, diarrhea
Less Common Serious Side Effects	Allergic reaction	None

Let's cover a few myths and facts about constipation so you know what should and shouldn't concern you as a parent. First, while one bowel movement per day is common, the normal range varies significantly. Some kids will go three times per day while others go just three times per week. Once your child drops below three per week, you're flirting with constipation. One per week and you've entered worrisome territory.

On the myth side, some people believe constipation makes the body absorb poisonous substances in stools. While regular bowel movements do aid in normal detoxification, there's no evidence that constipation leads to more severe conditions such as arthritis, asthma, or colon cancer.

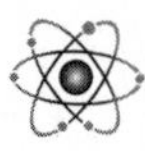

Science Says

Researchers at the Department of Pediatric Gastroenterology and Nutrition at the Emma Children's Hospital and Academic Medical Center in Amsterdam, Netherlands, conducted a systematic review of non-drug treatments for childhood constipation. Researchers reviewed nine major studies including 640 children. Researchers concluded that fiber supplements, among the non-drug treatments examined, showed the most positive evidence in improving the frequency and consistency of stools. That may also help explain why flaxseed powder—rich in fiber—is so effective.

Natural Selection

Flaxseed powder isn't the only flax option for constipation treatment. Oil from flaxseeds can act as a very effective stool softener as well; many brands like Barlean's are naturally flavored. Traditional Medicinals "Smooth Move" Tea (love the name!) made with natural senna may also help. If all else fails, there are always prunes and dates to get things moving.

Diarrhea

Diarrhea is a gastrointestinal condition that typically stems from a virus or dietary changes. Runny and frequent stools are the most common sign.

Diarrhea may also come from bacteria such as E. coli or salmonella, parasites from infected water, or contaminated food.

When diarrhea lasts longer than a few days or is particularly frequent in young children, the risk of dehydration is a concern. Oral rehydration may be required to replace lost fluids and electrolytes. Diarrhea may be accompanied by stomach pain, fever, nausea, vomiting, or decreased appetite.

Let's check out the treatment alternatives for diarrhea.

Diarrhea Side-by-Side Comparison

	Conventional Remedy	Treatment Alternative
Generic Treatment	Loperamide	Probiotics
Sample Brand Name Treatment	Imodium A-D Liquid	Florajen4Kids
How it works	Helps relieve symptoms of diarrhea such as stomach pain and runny stools.	Helps maintain a healthy immune system and achieve a balance of intestinal flora.
Dosage	Children under 6: ask a doctor; children ages 6-8: 15mL after loose stool and 7.5mL after subsequent loose stools, not exceeding 30mL in 24 hrs; children ages 9-11: 15mL after loose stool and 7.5mL after subsequent loose stools, not exceeding 45mL in 24 hrs; children ages 12+: 30mL after loose stool and 15mL after subsequent loose stools, not exceeding 60mL in 24 hrs.	One capsule daily, swallowed or sprinkled over food or into a beverage; consult a doctor prior to use in children under 2 years of age

	Conventional Remedy	Treatment Alternative
Active Ingredients	Loperamide hydrochloride	*Bifidobacterium lactis, Lactobacillus acidophilus, Bifidobacterium bifidum Bb-12, Lactobacillus rhamnosus*
Common Mild Side Effects	Drowsiness, dizziness, constipation, mild rash or itching, mild stomach pain	Gas
Less Common Serious Side Effects	Allergic reaction, stomach pain, worsening diarrhea, fever, sore throat, headache	Allergic reaction

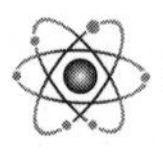

Science Says

Scientists at the Swansea University School of Medicine in the United Kingdom researched the effectiveness of probiotics in treating acute infectious diarrhea. Randomized controlled trials from 63 different studies (8,014 participants) evaluated probiotic agents versus a placebo. Of the 63 studies, 56 trials recruited infants and young children. Primary data points were the mean duration of diarrhea and stool frequency on both day two and four after intervention. Researchers discovered that, when used alongside rehydration therapy, probiotics appear to be safe and have clear beneficial impacts on shortening the duration and reducing stool frequency in acute infectious diarrhea.

Natural Selection

Beyond probiotics, you can also temporarily limit dairy products for your child during bouts of diarrhea to ease and heal the gastrointestinal system. Drinking warm chamomile tea may also soothe the gastrointestinal tract. Foods that bulk up the stool, like brown rice or bananas, are often recommended.

GERD/Reflux

"GERD" stands for "Gastro-Esophageal Reflux Disease," a fancy way of saying that food and drink are coming back up the wrong way from the stomach. GERD is more serious than the simple baby reflux we covered in Chapter 1.

The most common symptoms of GERD include coughing, "heartburn," gas, stomach pain, or vomiting shortly after consuming food.

Food allergies and sensitivities—and less commonly, medication reactions and neurological conditions—may also be to blame for these digestive problems.

Here's a look at the treatment options to consider if your child is suffering from GERD.

GERD/Reflux/Heartburn Side-by-Side Comparison

	Conventional Remedy	Treatment Alternative
Generic Treatment	Esomeprazole	Turmeric
Sample Brand Name Treatment	Nexium	Lee Silsby Enhansa
How it works	Nexium turns off acid-producing pumps in the stomach to decrease the amount of acid in the stomach.	Turmeric is a natural anti-inflammatory and aids in digestion.
Dosage	See package for dosage instructions; not for children under 1 year of age; ages 1-11: 10-20mg daily for up to 8 wks; ages 12-17: 20-40mg daily for up to 8 wks.	75-600mg per day per doctor's instructions

	Conventional Remedy	Treatment Alternative
Active Ingredients	Esomeprazole magnesium	Curcumin
Common Mild Side Effects	Headache, diarrhea, nausea, abdominal pain, somnolence	None
Less Common Serious Side Effects	Allergic reaction, chest pain, irregular heartbeat, fever, unusual bruising or bleeding	None

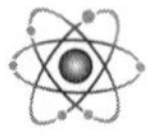

Science Says

Doctors at the Medical College of Wisconsin in Milwaukee studied the scientific rationale for curcumin (turmeric's active ingredient) as an anti-inflammatory agent in the gastrointestinal (GI) tract. Researchers concluded that curcumin inhibits the acid-induced expression of esophageal inflammation.

Natural Selection

A small amount of apple cider vinegar mixed into water and sipped can help ease heartburn and other reflux symptoms. Fennel seeds, consumed just after eating, can also help reduce reflux symptoms. Finally, aloe juice has been known to ease symptoms of gastroesophageal reflux.

Irritable Bowel Syndrome

Any ailment that has the word *irritable* in its title is worth tackling immediately. After all, we all know irritable kids cry, kick, scratch, act out, slam doors, and challenge your patience.

Irritable bowel syndrome, commonly referred to as IBS, is a digestive disorder that impacts the way the bowel system functions. Kids suffering from IBS find their stomach and colon simply don't function properly. This causes uncomfortable symptoms and a disruption of the bowel movement process.

✓ Good to Know

While 7-10 percent of the world's population suffers from irritable bowel syndrome, many are never diagnosed. That's millions of kids and parents assuming they're destined for irregular bowel movements for life, even though solutions are out there.

Common symptoms of IBS include pain in the stomach or abdomen, painful stools, gas, constipation, diarrhea, or bloating. These symptoms can be exacerbated by a poor diet, exposure to certain bacteria, medicines like antibiotics, and even stress.

Taking irritability out of your child's bowel movements means investigating and trying one of these conventional or natural treatment alternatives.

Irritable Bowel Syndrome Side-by-Side Comparison

	Conventional Remedy	Treatment Alternative
Generic Treatment	Dycyclomine	Enteric-coated peppermint oil
Sample Brand Name Treatment	Bentyl	Nature's Way Pepogest
How it works	Bentyl helps relax the muscles of the stomach and decreases stomach pain caused by IBS.	Pepogest helps soothe bowel disruptions and provides relief from gastrointestinal pain.*

	Conventional Remedy	Treatment Alternative
Dosage	Dosage determined by a doctor based on age, weight, and severity of IBS.	Consult a doctor before use in young children; take 1 softgel up to 3 times per day 30-60 minutes before a meal.
Active Ingredients	Dicyclomine hydrochloride	Peppermint oil, organic soybean oil
Common Mild Side Effects	Nausea, vomiting, drowsiness, dizziness, headache, constipation, decreased appetite, dry mouth, blurred vision, minor stomach pain, bloating	Heartburn
Less Common Serious Side Effects	Allergic reaction, confusion, irregular heartbeat, decreased urination, unusual changes in mood or behavior, trouble breathing, decreased coordination	None

**The enteric coating of the capsule prevents the oil from releasing in the stomach and causing irritation. Instead, the capsule can slowly dissolve in the small intestine where the oil can do its job without harm from inflammation.*

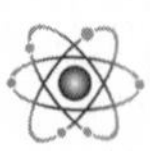

Science Says

Researchers at the University of Missouri-Columbia, Department of Child Health, Division of Pediatric Gastroenterology in Columbia, Missouri, studied the effectiveness of peppermint oil capsules in the treatment of irritable bowel syndrome in kids. In a randomized, double-blind controlled trial, 42 children with IBS were given peppermint oil capsules or a placebo. After two weeks, 75 percent of those kids receiving peppermint oil showed reduced severity of pain associated with IBS.

Natural Selection

Pure pear or prune juice can help the body produce healthy and regular stools. Also, an increase in the consumption of foods high in fiber (such as oats) helps to promote a healthy colon.

Probiotics introduce healthy bacteria to the gastrointestinal (GI) tract and can ease symptoms of IBS. Finally, drinking plenty of water each day (8 or more glasses) will help regulate bowel movements.

Motion Sickness

"Mommy, my tummy feels funny." It's one thing to hear this childhood complaint after dinner. It's quite another to hear this from the backseat of your shiny new car when the sign says, "Next rest area: 42 miles." Parents worldwide know an upset tummy is foreshadowing to a $500 interior car-cleaning bill. You might even sacrifice your designer pocketbook to catch the results of motion sickness and spare your car.

Motion sickness is a condition caused by the body's perception of movement. The inner ear transmits information regarding movement and balance to the brain. Misperceptions transmitted to the brain cause the symptoms of motion sickness.

Many forms of movement, the most common of which is driving in the car, can cause motion sickness. Kids may also feel motion sickness in a plane, boat, helicopter, or the mall carousel. Even sitting on the couch harmlessly watching TV can lead to motion sickness when the show has rapid and sudden movements.

Symptoms of motion sickness may include nausea, upset stomach, vomiting, increased saliva and sweating, fatigue, and dizziness. Before your kid plasters your leather seats with today's breakfast, you'll want to understand your treatment and prevention choices.

Motion Sickness Side-by-Side Comparison

	Conventional Remedy	Treatment Alternative
Generic Treatment	Dimenhydrinate	Ginger
Sample Brand Name Treatment	Dramamine Chewable Tablets (50mg, orange)	New Chapter GingerForce
How it works	Dramamine is an antiemetic that reduces symptoms of motion sickness such as nausea.	Ginger is a natural antiemetic that helps curb symptoms of motion sickness such as nausea.
Dosage	Not for children under 2 years of age; children ages 2-6: ¼-½ tablet every 6-8 hrs, not exceeding 1½ tablets in 24 hrs; children ages 6-11: ½-1 tablet every 6-8 hrs, not exceeding 3 tablets in 24 hrs; children ages 12+: 1-2 tablets every 4-6 hrs, not exceeding 8 tablets in 24 hrs.	Children old enough to swallow pills: 1 softgel daily, taken with food
Active Ingredients	Dimenhydrinate	Ginger hydroethanolic extract, ginger supercritical extract, rosemary supercritical extract
Common Mild Side Effects	Drowsiness;, dizziness, dry mouth, throat, or nose;, thickening mucus	None
Less Common Serious Side Effects	Allergic reaction, chest pain, convulsions, irregular heartbeat, fever, chills, wheezing, difficulty urinating, sore throat, decreased alertness	Rash due to allergic reaction, bloating, gas, heartburn, upset stomach

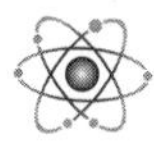

Science Says

At the Department of Internal Medicine, Division of Gastroenterology in Taipei, Taiwan, researchers studied the effects of ginger on motion sickness. They hypothesized that ginger ameliorates the nausea associated with motion sickness by preventing the development of gastric dysrhythmias. Researchers discovered that ginger prolonged the latency before nausea kicked in and also shortened recovery time after a motion sickness episode.

Natural Selection

If your child can't handle ginger in pill format, consider ginger tea or chewing on ginger candies such as GinGins to help reduce motion sickness symptoms. Homeopathic nux vomica or P6 acupressure may be helpful as well (see the next section on nausea/vomiting). Finally, teaching your child a distraction or relaxation strategy like guided imagery can be very productive.

Nausea/Vomiting

With all this talk about motion sickness and IBS, I'm starting to feel queasy myself—but we're not done yet. It's time to delve into nausea and vomiting. They go together like peanut butter and jelly. In other words, you rarely see one without the other as nausea is a frequent precursor of vomiting. Symptoms that may be associated with nausea and vomiting include decreased appetite, chills, sweating, headache, or sluggishness.

Vomiting plays an important role in body functioning. It rids the body of unpleasant stomach contents and helps expel toxins that are making the body ill. Nausea and vomiting may be brought on by an illness (often caused by a virus or bacteria), medication, allergic reaction, food poisoning, motion sickness, stress, eating too much, or even more serious health conditions.

Parental Guidance

"There is only one thing I can think of that I learned when I was a little girl and it has been wonderful for my family today. The use of water with lemon. You just take warm water (room temperature is fine) and squeeze a lemon into it. We usually use a strainer of some sort so the pits don't go into the cup but it is really that simple. It soothes the stomach, helps with digestion, and has just been a miracle in our house. Instead of reaching for the pink stuff we reach for the yellow."

—Rae Lyn, mother to a 5-year-old boy

A medical professional should see children with nausea and vomiting if symptoms persist beyond several hours or if accompanied by dehydration, diarrhea, or high fever. Here are the treatment options to consider before this ailment escalates to something requiring medical attention.

Nausea/Vomiting Side-by-Side Comparison

	Conventional Remedy	Treatment Alternative
Generic Treatment	Ondansetron	P6 Acupressure
Sample Brand Name Treatment	Zofran	Sea Bands
How it works	Zofran blocks receptors in the brain and gut that trigger nausea and vomiting.	Sea Bands apply pressure to the P6 acupressure point near the wrist to relieve symptoms of nausea and vomiting.

	Conventional Remedy	Treatment Alternative
Dosage	Use and dosage must be determined by a doctor; common doses: children ages 4-11: 4mg 3 times per day; children ages 12+: 8mg 2 times per day.	For use in children ages 3 or older: wear one Sea Band on each wrist with the button resting on the Nei-guan point (when placing the middle three fingers on the inside of the opposite wrist, the Nei-guan point is just under the index finger)
Active Ingredients	Ondansetron hydrochloride	N/A
Common Mild Side Effects	Constipation, diarrhea, fatigue, dizziness, headache	None
Less Common Serious Side Effects	Allergic reaction, chest or jaw pain, irregular heartbeat, chills, fever, seizure, fainting, difficulty urinating, changes in vision, muscle spasms	None

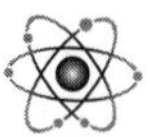

Science Says

The Department of Anesthesia and Intensive Care at the Chinese University of Hong Kong researched P6 wrist acupuncture effectiveness in postoperative nausea and vomiting (common complications after surgery and anesthesia). Nearly 5,000 participants were studied across 40 trials. Compared to a placebo treatment, those receiving acupoint stimulation showed significantly reduced nausea, vomiting, and need for rescue antiemetic medications. No serious adverse effects were noted.

Natural Selection

Quelling the feeling of nausea can be accomplished in multiple ways. First, pressing a cold compress to the forehead helps soothe the body. In the drinkable department, peach syrup can ease nausea, as can water with grated ginger mixed in or tea with warm water and clove. Mind-body techniques like hypnosis have been found effective for children with nausea and vomiting postoperatively or from medications like chemotherapy.

Recurrent Abdominal Pain

When you think about the word *recurrent* and your kids, wouldn't you love to hear phrases like "recurrent A+ in school" or "recurrent thank you" or "recurrent cleaning your room"? Unfortunately, many of those terms are better suited for the word *intermittent*. This section is about recurrent abdominal pain (or sometimes called functional abdominal pain), a specific type of bellyache with no single cause.

It's often hard to pinpoint the cause of abdominal pain because this area houses the digestive system (including the appendix) and key organs such as the kidneys, bladder, and liver. In girls, the uterus and ovaries also take up space in the abdominal area.

Parental Guidance

"My parents are Italian and a common stomach remedy in Italian households is fennel seed. I used to heat about ½ teaspoon of fennel seed in water for my daughter, strain it, and let her drink it slowly once it cooled. It was always good for infant gas, agita in older children and even nausea."

—Elise, mom to an 8-year-old girl

Recurrent abdominal pain is a unique condition defined as frequent and recurrent episodes of abdominal pain occurring over a three-month period. Symptoms can vary and include nausea, vomiting, diarrhea, or constipation, and often no physical cause is found. It is thought that these episodes can be aggravated by anxiety and may be accompanied by headache. Missed days of school can become problematic, so the more recurrent the abdominal pain for your child, the more important it becomes to consider one of the following treatment alternatives.

Recurrent Abdominal Pain Side-by-Side Comparison

	Conventional Remedy	Treatment Alternative
Generic Treatment	Amitriptyline	Hypnosis
Sample Brand Name Treatment	Elavil	Hypnotherapy
How it works	Small doses of the tricyclic antidepressant Elavil can help decrease the intensity and frequency of abdominal pain.	Hypnotherapy focuses on relaxing the body, including the stomach or digestive system, to reduce abdominal pain or symptoms of abdominal pain (such as diarrhea or constipation).
Dosage	Dosage must be determined by a medical professional based on the child's age, weight, and condition associated with abdominal pain.	Sessions should be with a trained hypnotherapist at a length and frequency determined by a medical professional.
Active Ingredients	Amitriptyline	N/A

	Conventional Remedy	Treatment Alternative
Common Mild Side Effects	Drowsiness, dizziness, constipation, dry mouth, heartburn, nausea, vomiting, blurred vision, headache, weakness, fatigue	None
Less Common Serious Side Effects	Allergic reaction, chest pain, confusion, muscle tremors, hair loss, nervousness, sweating, irregular heartbeat, changes in behavior, seizure, numbness, unusual bleeding or bruising, muscle spasms, suicidality	None

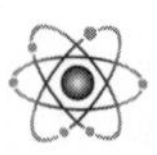

Science Says

The Department of Pediatrics at St. Antonius Hospital in The Netherlands studied hypnotherapy for children with functional abdominal pain. In all, 53 pediatric patients between the ages of 8 and 18 were randomized to either receive six hypnotherapy sessions over a three-month period or standard medical care and six sessions of supportive therapy. Researchers concluded that hypnotherapy was much more effective than standard care in reducing abdominal pain. Even one year later, at follow-up, treatment was deemed successful in 85 percent of the hypnotherapy group and only 25 percent of the standard medical therapy group.

Natural Selection

Other mind-body therapies, including yoga and meditation, may be helpful for recurrent abdominal pain. Massage and acupuncture have also been studied for this condition and help some children. Finally, probiotics also are worth trying to alleviate chronic, episodic abdominal pain.

Spotlight On: Mind-Body Medicine

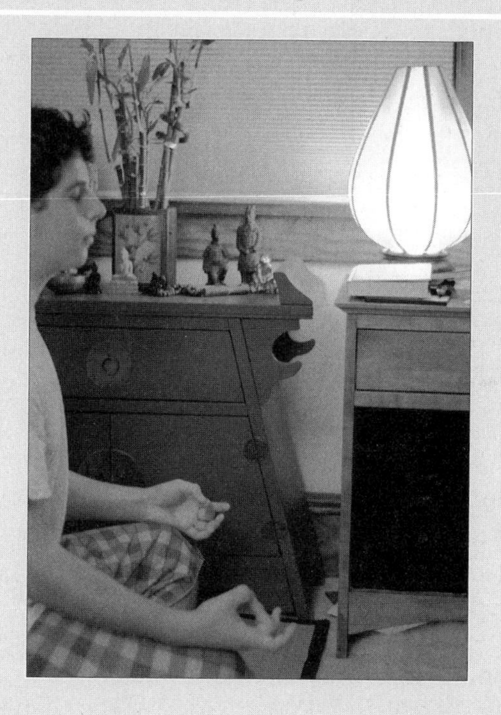

Meditation is one technique used in mind-body medicine.

Have you ever wondered why certain smells remind you of certain people? Or a song will jog memories of a long-ago love? These connections between mind and body are incredibly powerful, triggering surges of brain chemicals called neurotransmitters. Welcome to the world of mind-body medicine, a recognized form of healing by the NIH's National Center for Complementary and Alternative Medicine.

Many cultures have developed practices that harness the power of the mind-body connection with the purpose of calming the mind to improve bodily functioning and promote overall health. Many of these practices have been studied and found to have measurable physiological effects.

You've probably heard about the well-chronicled connection between stress and sickness. Everything from inflammation to depressed immune systems and major depression has been linked to mental stress. Well, the field of mind-body medicine capitalizes on the opposite association. It's based on the concept that positive emotions and thoughts can actually trigger beneficial physiological reactions.

It's worth checking out the scope of mind-body medicine techniques to see what resonates with your child. Examples include yoga, meditation, music therapy, biofeedback, hypnosis, and guided imagery. Entire books have been written on each, so start with simple searches for these terms and see what feels like the right fit for your child.

The beauty of these therapies is that they promote self-care and build confidence in a child's ability to heal himself. They are low-cost and portable, and children can develop mind-body stress coping skills to last them a lifetime.

Ultimately, it's worth investigating mind-body medicine as a complementary treatment approach for many of the conditions covered in this book.

7

Eating and Energy

"Making healthy choices when purchasing food today is more complicated than ever. Marketers know that parents want to buy nutritious choices, so if you are making your purchases based on the marketing messages on the front of the package, you are definitely misinformed! Go straight to the ingredients to determine if the foods contain natural or artificial ingredients—and of course, fruits and vegetables do not require packages! Engage your kids to do the same and the whole family will be at their best for energy and health. I have learned that if you eat the natural goodness from Mother Nature, she'll never let you down."

—Stacey Antine, MS, RD, founder of HealthBarn USA (www.healthbarnusa.com)

If you remember analogies from the SATs, you'll likely know that gas is to a car as food is to your child's body. Everything from participating in daily activities to keeping up with growth charts requires proper nutrition.

Unfortunately, certain ailments can interrupt your child's normal energy intake and growth projections. Everything from anemia and celiac disease to food allergies and high cholesterol can change how your child consumes food. Phrases like *fatigue* and *failure to thrive* enter the picture when nutrition is not up to snuff.

This chapter tackles the most common eating and energy ailments that strike babies and kids. If your child has been diagnosed with one of these ailments, read on to understand how you can make mealtime smooth sailing for years to come.

Anemia

When you think about oxygen, what comes to mind? Is it that precious air you breathe? Or maybe it's the key ingredient in water that mixes with hydrogen to refresh you on a warm summer day. Air and water sure are important, but neither has a monopoly on the need for oxygen. It turns out organs and tissues need oxygen to survive and thrive, too.

Red blood cells inside the body make sure organs and tissues receive enough oxygen to do their jobs. Anemia is a blood condition that results from the body having an insufficient amount of red blood cells, or hemoglobin, in the blood. When oxygen delivery is impaired, organs and tissue are simply unable to perform at their full potential.

Anemia results from a number of conditions, the most common of which is iron deficiency. Other causes include blood loss from an injury or internal bleeding, vitamin deficiencies, bone marrow disorders, kidney disease, or even sickle cell anemia (a condition where red blood cells are abnormally crescent-shaped and therefore deliver less oxygen to body tissue).

✓ **Good to Know**

Some types of anemia are hereditary, so your child can be affected from birth. Pregnant women are also at risk of anemia due to the increase in blood demand and nutritional needs during pregnancy.

Your child's most likely anemia symptom is fatigue due to a lack of oxygen in organs and tissues. Alongside fatigue, your child may also exhibit shortness of breath, dizziness, paleness, heart palpitations, and lightheadedness.

Once anemia is confirmed by your family pediatrician—typically by a simple in-office hemoglobin test—you'll want to check out these conventional remedies and treatment alternatives to pump up hemoglobin and get the oxygen flowing freely within your little one's body.

Anemia Side-by-Side Comparison

	Conventional Remedy	Treatment Alternative
Generic Treatment	Ferrous sulfate	Ferrous gluconate
Sample Brand Name Treatment	Feosol	Floradix Iron + Herbs
How it works	Feosol is an iron supplement that helps restore proper levels of iron in the body.	Floradix Iron + Herbs provides proper amounts of iron without unpleasant side effects. It is kosher and suitable for vegetarians.
Dosage	Children under 12: consult a doctor; children 12 years and older: take 1 tablet per day with water or juice on an empty stomach for maximum absorption.	Children 4-11: take 2 tsp once per day with food; children 12 years and older: take 2 tsp twice daily with food.
Active Ingredients	Ferrous sulfate	Ferrous gluconate, B vitamins, vitamin C
Common Mild Side Effects	Upset stomach, diarrhea, constipation, stomach cramps	None
Less Common Serious Side Effects	Allergic reaction	None

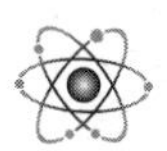

Science Says

Researchers at the Instituto Nacional de Salud Publica in Mexico studied the effect of adding ferrous gluconate and ascorbic acid (vitamin C) to milk sources for toddlers. Those children ingesting the vitamin- and mineral-fortified milk had significantly lower rates of anemia.

Natural Selection

There's a dietary supplement called lactoferrin—an antioxidant—that has been shown to reduce or eliminate iron deficiency (if this is the cause of your child's anemia). You can also look for pastas and cereals fortified with the right vitamins and minerals to combat anemia (again, iron is often the key lacking mineral, along with vitamin C, vitamin B_{12}, and folate). Even spinach (Popeye's favorite) can battle anemia, as it's rich in folate, iron, and vitamins. Finally, blackstrap molasses is extremely rich in iron and is a natural and vegetarian-friendly choice for curing anemic children.

Celiac Disease/Gluten Intolerance

Twenty years ago, very few people knew anything about gluten. In fact, it wouldn't have been surprising if someone confused it with a certain backside body part (the glutes)! Today, eating gluten-free is all the rage, and gluten-free products line the shelves of local health-conscious grocery stores. That's because celiac disease and gluten sensitivities have gone mainstream.

Celiac disease is an autoimmune condition that disrupts the natural digestion process. It makes it difficult for your child's body to digest any foods containing gluten.

Gluten is a protein found in grains such as wheat, rye, kamut, spelt, barley, and oats. It's a key ingredient in many of your kid's favorites including bagels, bread, muffins, pasta, and many pastries and desserts. While celiac disease and gluten are frequently linked together, it is possible to have gluten sensitivity without suffering from celiac disease.

The most common symptom of celiac disease or gluten sensitivity is abdominal pain after eating foods rich in wheat. This pain may also lead to gas, bloating, diarrhea, and constipation.

Parental Guidance

"When I found out about my own gluten intolerance I was crushed. All of my favorites like pasta, bread, and pastries were on the brink of elimination. My child too started showing signs of difficulty processing gluten. Luckily we found we're not alone and food companies galore now produce gluten-free alternatives to some of our favorites. Thankfully we can still enjoy banana pancakes every Sunday morning. There's no wheat but the taste doesn't miss a beat!"

—Carol, loving mother to 5-year-old Gabe and 2-year-old Sienna

If your child has been diagnosed with celiac disease or gluten sensitivity, it's unfortunately a chronic condition. However, you can help your child keep the symptoms at bay by following a gluten-free diet and complementing that strategy with treatment alternatives such as probiotics as discussed here. For those with celiac disease (as opposed to only a gluten sensitivity), it is imperative to follow a gluten-free diet.

Celiac Disease/Gluten Intolerance Side-by-Side Comparison

	Conventional Remedy	Treatment Alternative
Generic Treatment	Gluten-free diet	Probiotics
Sample Brand Name Treatment	N/A	VSL#3 (in addition to a gluten-free diet)
How it works	Removing gluten from the diet will help eliminate symptoms of celiac disease.	VSL#3 contains healthy bacteria that works in conjunction with the GI tract to form a barrier against harmful bacteria and substances that cause inflammation.

	Conventional Remedy	Treatment Alternative
Dosage	N/A	Dosage for children and infants is dependent upon age, weight, and average number of bowel movements per day.
Active Ingredients	N/A	Lactic acid bacteria
Common Mild Side Effects	N/A	Mild bloating
Less Common Serious Side Effects	N/A	None

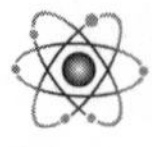

Science Says

Researchers at the University of Bari in Italy studied the effectiveness of VSL#3 probiotics in decreasing the toxicity of wheat flour from fermentation. Researchers found VSL#3 played an important role in producing predigested and tolerated gliadins, which in turn helped with the palatability of gluten-free products. Researchers at the Department of Gastroenterology and Hepatology at the University Hospital of Santiago de Compostela in Spain went a step further and examined enzyme replacement therapy for those suffering from celiac disease. The study demonstrated extra support from dietary enzymes for celiacs.

Natural Selection

Klaire Vital-Zymes can provide enzyme support for children with digestive issues, including celiac disease. While this product may make the digestion process easier, it's important to note that this does not replace the benefits of a gluten-free diet. However, it may be helpful as an add-on for any gut inflammation your child experiences. You can also go the herbal route with your child to ameliorate celiac disease and gluten sensitivity issues. Turmeric and chamomile are two herbs that can help with inflammation and cramping.

Failure to Thrive

You've likely seen hundreds of baby announcements in your day. The email or announcement card might say something like, "We're excited to announce the birth of our baby boy, Joey! Weight: 7 pounds; length: 20 inches." It's a cute reminder of just how small babies are when they enter the world. From there you go back to your latte and work to-do list, never to think of that baby's height and weight again.

For parents of children who fail to thrive, height and weight become all-too-important measurements. The failure to thrive label is given to children, most commonly babies and toddlers, whose height and weight are significantly below the curve and are not increasing at the right rate for age. The average and typical measurements can be found on standardized growth charts based on gender and age. Pediatricians commonly keep these records as your child grows.

✓ Good to Know

The average birth weight of a full-term newborn is 7.5 pounds. The average length is around 18 to 20 inches. By age 3, girls are typically 26 to 39 pounds and 35 to 40 inches in length while boys are, on average, 27 to 39 pounds and 36 to 41 inches tall. Of course, growth is based on many factors, including genetics and nutrition.

The most common causes of failure to thrive include premature birth, poor nutrition, aversions to nutritious food and drink, or even childhood stress (e.g., an unhappy home). Your pediatrician is in the best position to check your child's height and weight to see where she fits on the growth scale.

Less common causes can also lead to failure to thrive. These include medical conditions like gastrointestinal and endocrine disorders. If your child is in the lowest percentiles for height and/or weight, you'll want to read this section closely for treatment alternatives.

Failure to Thrive Side-by-Side Comparison

	Conventional Remedy	Treatment Alternative
Generic Treatment	Milk protein concentrate	Organic cow's milk with vitamins and minerals
Sample Brand Name Treatment	Pediasure (vanilla)	Pediasmart (vanilla)
How it works	Pediasure is a gluten- free and kosher source of nutrition for kids needing additional nutrition.	Pediasmart is an organic nutritional supplement containing vitamins and minerals. It works well for those with lactose intolerance, those with celiac disease, and those who require a kosher diet; there is also a soy-based version for those with cow's milk allergies.
Dosage	Drink 1-3 bottles per day or follow a doctor's instructions.	For children ages 1-13: 8 oz per serving 1-3 times per day or as advised by a doctor.
Active Ingredients	Water, sugar, corn maltodextrin, milk protein concentrate, high oleic safflower oil, soy oil, whey protein concentrate, medium-chain triglycerides	Organic rice oligodextrin, organic evaporated cane syrup, organic lactose-free milk protein concentrate, organic high oleic sunflower oil, safflower oil, organic soybean oil, organic coconut oil, organic vanilla
Common Mild Side Effects	None	None
Less Common Serious Side Effects	None	None

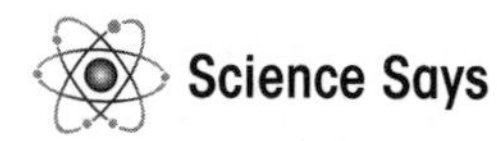

Science Says

Getting calories into your child is critical in battling a failure to thrive. However, many choices contain high fructose corn syrup (HFCS), and this can lead to obesity and related metabolic disorders like diabetes. Researchers at the Pennington Biomedical Research Center at Louisiana State University found a connection between HFCS in foods and beverages and the obesity epidemic. Researchers concluded that patterns from the U.S. Department of Agriculture food consumption tables over a 30-year period mirrored the rise in obesity in America.

Natural Selection

Dr. Rosen has his own homegrown recipe for rice milk smoothies, a good source of protein and calcium to help a baby or child get necessary nutrition for growth. This recipe is especially well suited for kids with milk and soy allergies or sensitivities. Simply combine 6 ounces of rice milk, ½ tablespoon of rice protein powder, and 1 teaspoon of flaxseed powder with additional fruits (and vegetables if you dare) for flavoring. Almond milk is a good low-carb substitute for those not allergic to tree nuts. It's rich in calcium; you can add organic almond butter for a healthy fat boost.

Otherwise, focus on meals and snacks that are high in calories based on healthy fats, carbohydrates, and proteins.

Fatigue

Children are known for their endless expendable energy, so prolonged fatigue may be cause for concern. Fatigue is often a symptom of illness, such as a cold or a case of the flu. Exhaustion and fatigue are also side effects of many medications taken for cold, flu, or allergies.

Fatigue may also be a natural result of a child's growth spurt. A child may require more sleep if he or she is in the midst of growing. Or it can be an indication of a medical condition, as it is a key symptom for conditions such as anemia, celiac disease, and mononucleosis.

For general fatigue unrelated to a medical condition, many parents rely on commercial nutrition drinks such as PediaSure and BOOST. However, you might want an alternative if either the sugar content or tolerance of lactose is an issue so we've provided one in the table. Also worthy of note here is more and more children (often unbeknownst to parents) are unfortunately turning to caffeinated beverages like Red Bull for energy. The American Academy of Pediatrics specifically cautions against the use of energy drinks in children, noting, "Energy drinks contain substances not found in sports drinks that act as stimulants, such as caffeine, guarana and taurine. Caffeine—by far the most popular stimulant—has been linked to a number of harmful health effects in children, including effects on the developing neurologic and cardiovascular systems."

Fatigue Side-by-Side Comparison

	Conventional Remedy	Treatment Alternative
Generic Treatment	Milk, sugar, added vitamins	Carnitine, CoQ10, quercetin
Sample Brand Name Treatment	BOOST Kid Essentials	Prothera MitoThera
How it works	Milk and sugar provide ready-to-use energy for the body.	Prothera MitoThera is a natural source of energy for those experiencing fatigue, providing nutrients and energy substrates.
Dosage	One serving as needed.	Take two tablets daily with food.

	Conventional Remedy	Treatment Alternative
Active Ingredients	Sucrose, fructose, sodium caseinate	Magnesium, sodium, coenzyme Q10, N-acetyl-l-cysteine USP, alpha-lipoic acid, creatine, monohydrate, malic acid, quercetin, red grape extract, sodium succinate, ecithin, phoshatidylcholine
Common Mild Side Effects	Nausea, gas, bloating, cramps (lactose intolerance)	None
Less Common Serious Side Effects	None	None

Science Says

Researchers at the Key Laboratory of General Administration of Sport in Shanghai, China, found nutrients like coenzyme Q10 and carnitine stimulate performance in exhaustively exercised rats. Their findings suggest mitochondrial nutrients may play a role in the enhancement of physical performance and fatigue recovery. In a separate study, researchers at the Division of Applied Physiology at the University of South Carolina studied the dietary flavonoid quercetin. They found that quercetin successfully increased VO_2max, the maximum capacity of a human body to transport and use oxygen while exercising.

Natural Selection

Omega-3 fatty acids, found in salmon and flaxseeds, for example, help provide the body with extra energy in the form of healthy fats. Your child can also consume omega-3s in supplement form. Many of the

B vitamins are considered "energy" boosters, including B_1, B_2, B_3, B_6, and B_{12}. These are commonly combined in a vitamin B-complex supplement. Together omega-3s and B vitamins also support mitochondrial metabolism.

Food Allergies

Between three square meals and snacking, we sure do eat a lot during the day. Add the pre-bedtime noshing and many kids are eating six or seven times per day. For most kids, food concerns focus on eating too much or too little, or too much of the wrong things and too little of healthy alternatives. This is not the chief concern for kids with food allergies. One consumption mistake can potentially be life-threatening for severe allergy sufferers.

We don't typically expect peanuts, seafood, and other common food allergens to start a fight inside our child's body. However, when a child suffers from a food allergy, the body misidentifies the food as something foreign and harmful. The immune system kicks into high gear and creates symptoms ranging from mild to life-threatening. These reactions run the gamut from diarrhea and rashes to throat swelling and difficulty breathing. Unfortunately, more and more children are being diagnosed with food allergies than ever before.

Parental Guidance

"My son suffered seafood and chicken allergies throughout his childhood. Luckily, he outgrew the chicken allergy, but seafood remains a challenge. We found the most effective game plan was prevention, simply teaching my son to ask waiters and chefs about ingredients before consuming anything unusual. It's amazing how seafood finds its way into sauces, pasta dishes, and even dips."

—Janis, mother to lifelong seafood-allergy-suffering son

Among the most common food allergies are peanuts, tree nuts, gluten, seafood, cow's milk, soy, and eggs. The challenge goes beyond simply your child's avoidance of these foods. In many cases, severe allergy sufferers react when consuming otherwise harmless foods prepared with or near ingredients that cause allergic reactions. This issue in part led to changing food label rules requiring companies to list other common allergens (e.g., peanuts) produced in shared facilities and factories. In cases of children with severe allergies, it's important to carry ready-to-use injections of epinephrine like an EpiPen. This provides a first-line treatment for emergency allergic reactions (anaphylaxis).

While your child may simply outgrow a food allergy with age, you can also check out these complementary treatment options while waiting to see if adulthood is the ultimate cure. Of course, whatever treatment option you choose, teaching your child to avoid those foods causing allergic reactions should be the first line of defense.

Science Says

Researchers at the Skin and Allergy Hospital at the University of Helsinki in Finland studied the connection between probiotics and development of food allergies in babies. Scientists studied a cohort of 327 allergy-prone infants receiving either probiotics or a placebo to see how gut immune markers change with respect to the development of eczema, food allergies, asthma, and rhinitis. Those ingesting probiotics, compared with controls, had significantly positive changes in immune markers indicating reduced risk of food allergies. Also, infants born via C-section and treated with probiotics were less likely to have allergic disorders than controls even at 5 years of age.

Food Allergies Side-by-Side Comparison

	Conventional Remedy	Treatment Alternative
Generic Treatment	Diphenhydramine	Probiotics
Sample Brand Name Treatment	Benadryl Allergy UltraTab Tablets	Klaire Ther-Biotic Infant
How it works	The active ingredient temporarily relieves allergic symptoms including runny nose, sneezing, watery eyes, and itchy throat.	This is a hypo-allergenic blend that provides metabolic and intestinal support to the body.
Dosage	Under 6 years: don't use; 6-12 years: 1 tablet every 4-6 hrs.; over 12 years: 1-2 tablets every 4-6 hrs.	¼ tsp daily with food, after consulting with a medical professional
Active Ingredients	Diphenhydramine HCl	Probiotic blend, *lactobacillus* species, *Lactobacillus rhamnosus, Lactobacillus casei, Lactobacillus paracasei, Lactobacillus gasseri, Lactobacillus saliverius, bifidobacterium* species, *Bifidobacterium bifidum, Bifidobacterium infantis, Bifidobacterium lactis, Bifidobacterium longum, Bifidobacterium breve*
Common Mild Side Effects	Drowsiness, dizziness, headache, nausea, upset stomach, constipation, diarrhea, excitability, loss of appetite, nervousness, anxiety, trouble sleeping, vomiting, weakness	None

	Conventional Remedy	Treatment Alternative
Less Common Serious Side Effects	Difficulty urinating, severe allergic reaction, irregular heartbeat, mood changes, hallucinations, seizures, tremor, vision changes, yellowing of skin or eyes	None

Natural Selection

When expectant mothers take prenatal probiotics, studies have demonstrated a reduction in allergic disorders in their children even as late as seven years later. The timing of introducing foods into a child's diet may also prevent certain food allergies and intolerances. While this point is hotly debated, a common example includes waiting to introduce cow's milk until age 1. For some infants at high risk for development of food allergies, it may be prudent to wait until a year or later to introduce highly allergenic foods like peanuts or shellfish. Avoidance of known food allergens is the safest way to avoid serious problems.

High Cholesterol

We don't typically see high cholesterol commercials aimed at little kids. It's commonly thought to be an ailment for adults with high blood pressure, obesity, and other heart-related symptoms. Still, it is possible for children to have higher-than-normal cholesterol. More children and teens are at risk due to complications of obesity. Tackling metabolic concerns while young is the best way to avoid a lifelong battle with cholesterol.

There are different types of cholesterol in the human body. We still are discovering new facts about the harmful and protective effects of these different types. In very simple terms that do not reflect the complex nature of how lipids (fats) impact our risk for disease, here's what we do know. Low-density lipoproteins (LDL) are the harmful, artery-clogging type, while high-density lipoproteins (HDL) are thought to be heart-protective. If your child has too much LDL and not enough HDL, he is at higher risk to build up plaque on his arteries. This plaque buildup combined with inflammation can ultimately lead to heart attacks and strokes.

A simple blood test can determine your child's cholesterol level. Overweight children and those with a family history of high cholesterol are most at risk for elevated readings. Exercise and improved diet are common recommendations to improve cholesterol numbers, as are the following conventional and natural treatment alternatives.

High Cholesterol Side-by-Side Comparison

	Conventional Remedy	Treatment Alternative
Generic Treatment	Statins	Fish oil
Sample Brand Name Treatment	Lipitor	Nordic Naturals ProOmega
How it works	Lipitor is a statin that lowers cholesterol and triglycerides.	ProOmega provides high levels of the omega-3 fatty acids EPA and DHA, which can help reduce cholesterol.
Dosage	Dosage of Lipitor must be determined by a doctor.	1-2 capsules daily as advised by a doctor
Active Ingredients	Atorvastatin calcium	Purified deep sea fish oil
Common Mild Side Effects	Fatigue, diarrhea, upset stomach, muscle or joint pain	Mild burping

	Conventional Remedy	Treatment Alternative
Less Common Serious Side Effects	Muscle problems, kidney failure, liver problems, allergic reaction	None

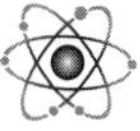

Science Says

Researchers at the Telethon Institute for Child Health Research at the University of Western Australia studied how omega-3s correlate with healthier food consumption in children and with a reduced risk of cardiovascular disease in adolescent boys. In the study, over 1,300 boys, ages 13 to 15, were tracked. Researchers found a positive correlation between omega-3 fatty acid concentrations in kids and intake of fish and whole grains. The reverse was true for adolescents with high consumption of soft drinks and unhealthy snack foods.

Natural Selection

Beyond exercise, omega-3s, and healthier eating, artichoke leaf extract may help lower LDL cholesterol levels. Red yeast rice is also thought to lower cholesterol and the risk of cardiac disease. Finally, garlic consumption is associated with lower LDL levels.

Spotlight On: Vitamins and Supplements

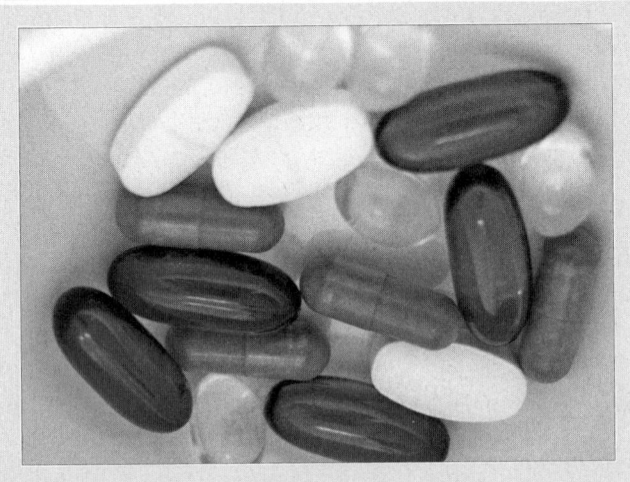

Vitamins and supplements can enhance attention.

The safest and most effective way to consume vitamins and minerals is from an organic, whole foods diet rich in fruits and vegetables. Though there is a debate about ideal amounts of specific vitamins and minerals needed for optimal health, ensuring regular intake of healthy nutrients is crucial. Under certain conditions, it's not always possible to obtain adequate levels of all nutrients, as in those with food allergies and gastrointestinal disorders.

It turns out the benefits of adequate vitamins and minerals may stretch beyond bodily health. Optimal nutrient levels are needed for maximum cognitive functioning. Researchers at the Human Cognitive Neuroscience Unit at Northumbria University in the United Kingdom discovered positive cognitive and mood effects for healthy children receiving 12-week supplementation of multivitamins and minerals.

Scientists studied 81 healthy children ranging in age from 8 to 14 years. The children were tested for cognitive performance and general mood prior to supplementation, then again after 12 weeks of supplementation. Interim assessments were also done at four and eight weeks during the trial. Among the functions tested were attention, memory, spatial skills, and mood. The children receiving the supplements showed improved performance in attention-based tasks, while less conclusive evidence was discovered for mood enhancement. Still, as a parent, it's nice to know that a daily multivitamin may help your child pay better attention in school. Combined with exercise and adequate rest, nutrition plays a key role in children's physical and mental health.

8

Midsection Maladies

"There are multiple complementary therapies that have been used for common urinary ailments. Fluids, good voiding patterns, treating underlying constipation, probiotics, mind-body therapies (such as hypnosis, guided imagery, and biofeedback), and some nutritional supplements (cranberry and blueberry extracts in particular) have been shown to be beneficial."

—Matthew Hand, DO, Director, Pediatric Nephrology and Integrative Medicine, New Hampshire's Hospital for Children

Arms and legs get so much publicity. Must be their abilities to wave, shake hands, jump, do splits, and climb. The midsection keeps it all together yet gets little fanfare. All of that changes when the ailments presented in this chapter surface. Everything from bed-wetting and kidney stones to menstrual cramps and urinary tract infections can grind jumping and splits to a halt.

If your child has one of these midsection maladies, you'll want to read this section closely to understand the conventional remedies and treatment alternatives available. You'll also be surprised to find out some unexpected ailments, such as kidney stones, are creeping into the toddler years.

Ultimately, let's work together in this chapter to get arms and legs back in the limelight. We want your kid's childhood defined by running, jumping, and clapping, not midsection maladies. Here's to a healthy midsection, free of ailments, keeping a low profile.

Bed-wetting

Every Wednesday morning, you religiously change the bed sheets in your child's bedroom. You've got a routine down. First it's breakfast for the little one, then it's playtime while you make the quick sheet swap. Unfortunately, something has disrupted your weekly routine. Bed-wetting has turned a weekly chore into a daily one. You're running out of clean bed sheets—and patience, too.

Transitioning from diapers to underwear takes time. That's why several successful books have been written on potty training. While accidents can happen anytime, it's the nighttime that's trickier. You can't exactly tell your sleeping toddler to let you know when something is coming.

Bed-wetting can also go beyond just potty training. Emotional or physical stress, environmental changes (e.g., a new house), or even bladder infections can all lead to bed-wetting. Some researchers even believe it's hereditary—not that you'll be anxious to ask your spouse if he was a bed-wetter! Additionally, temporary bed-wetting may occur when your child is fighting off illness like the common cold.

The good news is that most kids outgrow bed-wetting as they gain better control over their bladders. However, if you can't wait for your little one's bladder to get trained, check out these treatment alternatives. Your bed sheets will thank you for the effort.

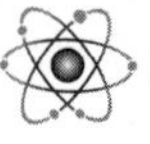

Science Says

In 1985, SD Edwards and HI van der Spuy published some of the earliest trials on the effectiveness of hypnotherapy in treating bed-wetting. In their research, 48 boys, ages 8 to 13, were studied over six months. With one-hour weekly sessions, test subjects showed significant decreases in bed-wetting episodes compared to a control group. Another study from India found hypnotherapy more effective than a prescription drug (imipramine) to treat nocturnal enuresis (nighttime wetting) over a nine-month period.

Bed-wetting Side-by-Side Comparison

	Conventional Remedy	Treatment Alternative
Generic Treatment	Desmopressin	Hypnosis
Sample Brand Name Treatment	DDAVP	N/A
How it works	DDVAP acts as a hormone and helps decrease thirst and keep bed-wetting to a minimum by controlling the production of urine.	Hypnosis helps discourage bed-wetting by placing the body in a relaxed state and suggesting an alternate behavior, such as responding to a full bladder while asleep the same way one would respond to a full bladder while awake.
Dosage	Dosage is determined by a doctor based on age and weight; common dose is one pill daily before bed.	Hypnosis sessions should be determined by a practitioner. Duration of treatment is based upon the individual.
Active Ingredients	Desmopressin acetate	N/A
Common Mild Side Effects	Diarrhea, changes in thought process	None
Less Common Serious Side Effects	Nausea, vomiting, loss of appetite, headache, irritability, fatigue, hallucinations, restlessness, weight gain, weakness, decreased appetite, allergic reaction	None

Natural Selection

Many parents institute a middle-of-the-night trip to the bathroom to reduce bed-wetting during potty training. Sure, it's a little lost sleep for parent and child, but you make up the time not having to change the sheets the next morning. Limiting fluids after dinner is another time-tested approach. Alternatively, you can have your child wear a pad with built-in alarm sensors. The sensors emit a noise or vibration whenever wetness is detected. This can help your little one become aware of an impending accident. Finally, Blue Poppy's Dry Nites is a traditional Chinese medicine formula that may treat bed-wetting by correcting, as the manufacturer notes, "a combination of lung, spleen, and kidney qi vacuity which is the most commonly seen pattern of pediatric bed-wetting." Qi is defined in Chinese medicine as a form of energy or life-force that flows in and out of us. Treatments in Chinese medicines, including herbals, acupuncture, and massage, can be directed at increasing or decreasing the flow of qi along meridians (for more information on acupuncture, see Chapter 12).

Kidney Stones

The Rolling Stones made "(I Can't Get No) Satisfaction" famous. Perhaps this song should have instead been associated with kidney stones. Stemming from an imbalance in urine mineral concentration, kidney stones range from somewhat painful to worst-pain-in-your-life painful.

Your child's urine normally contains water, minerals, and acids, among other components. When the balance is off, crystals may form and turn into kidney stones. In many cases, these crystals—particularly when small in size—are passed harmlessly during urination. Larger stones may require medical attention.

✓ Good to Know

Kidney stones are on the rise in kids. The two biggest risk factors are not drinking enough fluids and eating too much salt. Both increase the amount of calcium and oxalate in the urine that bind together into kidney stones. In fact, more than half of all pediatric kidney stone cases can be tied back to oxalate binding to calcium in the urine.

While many kidney stones can be attributed to changing calcium levels in the urine, this is not the only cause. Dehydration and urinary tract infections can lead to kidney stones, too.

The most common kidney stone symptoms include pain when urinating; brown or pink urine; frequent urination urges; and pain in the lower back, groin, or abdomen. Blood may also appear in the urine. Regardless of the cause or specific symptoms, you'll want to learn about your treatment options.

Kidney Stones Side-by-Side Comparison

	Conventional Remedy	Treatment Alternative
Generic Treatment	Lithotripsy	Lemon juice in water
Sample Brand Name Treatment	N/A	N/A
How it works	Lithotripsy is the physical destruction of kidney stones through non-invasive shock waves.	A combination of lemon juice and water helps to raise pH levels in urine, which helps prevent kidney stones from developing.
Dosage	N/A	Juice from one lemon mixed with three cups of water and consumed once per day or as needed
Active Ingredients	N/A	Lemon, water

	Conventional Remedy	Treatment Alternative
Common Mild Side Effects	Localized pain or discomfort, blood in the urine, infection	Heartburn
Less Common Serious Side Effects	Allergic reaction, chest pain, convulsions, irregular heartbeat, fever, chills, wheezing, difficulty urinating, sore throat, decreased alertness, renal damage	None

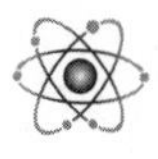

Science Says

Researchers at Unita Complessa di Urologia in Treviso, Italy, studied urinary alkalization as it relates to kidney stone formation. Scientists determined three major factors that impact the likelihood of developing kidney stones—the excretion of uric acid, the volume of urine in relation to uric acid concentration, and low urinary pH. Of the three, urinary pH is the most important factor for stone formation. Lemon juice has been shown to help increase urinary pH, thereby decreasing the likelihood of stones while also helping to dissolve existing stones.

Natural Selection

Diet plays a key role in limiting stones or keeping them at bay entirely. Different types of stones—uric acid, calcium oxalate, etc.—respond to different dietary restrictions. Above all else, fluids are key. Drinking at least 8 to 10 glasses of water per day deters kidney stones from forming. If stones still develop, consider a mixture of olive oil and lemon juice together to help dissolve or pass a kidney stone. Eating black cherries or drinking cherry juice has been helpful to prevent the development of some kinds of kidney stones.

Labial Adhesions

Parents worry about everything when it comes to their kids' private parts. Often it's focused on diaper rash and stool irregularities. Sometimes the ailment of concern—for girls—is a labial adhesion.

This condition, which affects up to 2 percent of young girls, occurs when the two inner lips of the vagina merge together. The adhesion may be partial, impacting only a portion of the labia minora. In more severe cases, the entire length of the labia minora can adhere together.

Labial adhesions are thought to be caused by new tissue growth that inadvertently fuses together the vagina's inner lips. This new tissue that forms may be the result of skin healing from inflammation or irritation (e.g., after a soiled diaper). Additionally, low levels of estrogen may cause the labia minora to adhere together.

When suffering a labial adhesion, your daughter may experience difficulty urinating and pain when the legs are spread for a diaper change. A bladder or urinary tract infection may also develop from an adhesion if the urine is not able to properly pass through the urethra. Here are the conventional remedies and treatment alternatives available.

Labial Adhesions Side-by-Side Comparison

	Conventional Remedy	Treatment Alternative
Generic Treatment	Estrogen	Calendula
Sample Brand Name Treatment	Premarin cream	Weleda Calendula
How it works	Premarin promotes a gradual separation of the labia minora, which resolves labial adhesion.	This ointment helps moisturize, heal, and soothe skin problems such as irritation and damage associated with labial adhesion.

	Conventional Remedy	Treatment Alternative
Dosage	Apply a pea-sized amount of Premarin topically 2 times per day for 2 weeks or as directed by a doctor.	Apply ointment to the affected area 3-4 times per day.
Active Ingredients	Conjugated estrogens (mixture of estrogen hormones)	*Calendula officinalis*
Common Mild Side Effects	Headache, abdominal pain, joint or back pain, bloating, diarrhea, dizziness, breast tenderness, hair loss	None
Less Common Serious Side Effects	Liver damage, stroke, blood clots, lumps in the breast, tightness in the chest, vaginal itching or redness, bleeding, numbness, shortness of breath, changes in vision	None

Science Says

According to the Natural Standard Research Collaboration, animal-based studies have shown that topical application of calendula extracts help reduce inflammation. This holds true in a wide variety of skin irritations including sunburn, eczema, and psoriasis. Further, the Natural Comprehensive Medicines Database notes that the anti-inflammatory properties of calendula stem from the presence of faradiol esters in the flowers.

Natural Selection

In minor cases, labial adhesions will typically resolve with no treatment whatsoever. Typically, this ailment will rarely go beyond toddler years. If the condition persists or is bothersome, another treatment alternative is the topical application of coconut oil or flaxseed oil to help lubricate the tissue in the labial region.

Menstrual Cramps

We're midway through the book and have finally arrived at an ailment parents of young children (or boys only) may skip. Sure, you can read about menstrual cramps if you're eager for foreshadowing on future ailments. I'm guessing you have enough to worry about just chasing your toddler and keeping her fingers out of sockets.

Menstrual cramps, technically called dysmenorrhea, are crampy pains that coincide with female menstruation. Pain can vary from slight to debilitating and usually affects the lower back, stomach, and pelvic area.

The cramps stem from muscle contractions assisting in the monthly shedding of the inner lining of the uterus. The cramps felt are actually uterine contractions, usually—but not always—much milder than those felt at childbirth.

✓ Good to Know

Over the course of her lifetime, the average woman will spend approximately 3,500 days menstruating. This time period ends with menopause. Human females are not the only mammals that make the transition; both elephants and humpback whales also undergo menopause.

Beyond midsection pain, the most common symptoms accompanying menstrual cramps include headache, nausea, diarrhea, or constipation. These symptoms are usually confined to the first few days of menstruation. The following treatment options may help your teenage daughter cope with the symptoms.

Menstrual Cramps Side-by-Side Comparison

	Conventional Remedy	Treatment Alternative
Generic Treatment	Naprosyn	Vitamin B_1
Sample Brand Name Treatment	Anaprox	BlueBonnet Vitamin B_1
How it works	Anaprox helps relieve pain and tenderness caused by menstrual cramps for those with extreme pain during the menstrual cycle.	Vitamin B_1 helps provide significant relief of menstrual symptoms such as cramping when taken in supplement form.
Dosage	Dosage must be determined by a medical professional based on age, weight, and severity of menstrual cramps.	Take one capsule daily as directed by a doctor.
Active Ingredients	Naproxen sodium	Vitamin B_1 (thiamine)
Common Mild Side Effects	Heartburn, stomach pain, nausea, headache, fatigue, dizziness, constipation, itching, bloating, shortness of breath	None
Less Common Serious Side Effects	Allergic reaction, shortness of breath, chest pain, slurred speech, internal bleeding, bloody nose, vomiting that contains blood, bloody stools, kidney failure, liver damage	None

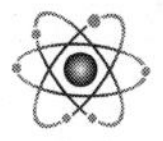

Science Says

Researchers at the Department of Obstetrics and Gynecology at the National Women's Hospital in Auckland, New Zealand, studied both herbal and dietary therapies for menstrual cramps. In various studies, the lead researchers found both vitamin B_1 and magnesium to be promising treatments for dysmenorrhea. The recommended dosage for vitamin B_1 is 100mg daily. More research is needed to determine the best daily dosage for magnesium.

Natural Selection

Aviva Romm, MD (also a noted herbalist and midwife; www.avivaromm.com), suggests a combination of herbal liquid extracts containing equal parts of the herbs cramp bark and ginger root to treat menstrual cramps. Take 2-3 mL (about ½ measured teaspoon) every 2-4 hours during cramps. The "cramp bark" relaxes the cramps as does ginger while also acting as a mild anti-inflammatory.

Limiting caffeine can also provide menstrual cramp relief, as can replacing caffeinated drinks with raspberry or chamomile tea to soothe the uterine nervous system. Taking fish oil supplements may also reduce cramping by decreasing bodily levels of prostaglandin, a hormone that is partially responsible for cramps. In more severe cases, consider acupuncture or acupressure, particularly focused on a specific acupoint on the inner ankle. This spot, known as "Spleen 6," is thought to reduce menstrual cramping sensations.

Urinary Tract Infection

Earlier in this chapter, we covered how labial adhesions may lead to urinary tract infections (UTIs). Whether caused by adhesions or other factors, urinary tract infections occur when bacteria enters the urinary tract, contaminating a previously sterile part of the body. Starting at the urethra, the infection can travel up the urinary tract past the bladder and up to the kidneys if left untreated.

Beyond labial adhesions, urinary tract infections may be associated with poor toileting hygiene and improper cleaning after urination or bowel movements. Younger children are susceptible to urinary tract infections because they may not wipe properly after going to the bathroom. Some babies are born with vesicoureteral reflux, meaning regurgitation of urine back up the ureters to the kidney during voiding; this condition may predispose these babies to urinary tract infections.

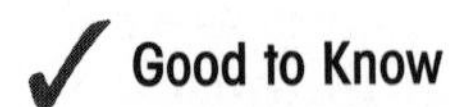

Most folks associate urinary tract infections with girls. By the age of 5, approximately 8 percent of girls have had at least 1 UTI. However, boys may experience the ailment, too, as 1 to 2 percent of boys under 5 have also had at least 1 UTI. While relatively rare in boys without urinary reflux, UTIs may be somewhat more common in uncircumcised boys.

Diabetic children, those with kidney problems, and kids with poorly functioning bladders are at higher risk for urinary tract infections. Common symptoms include pain when urinating, cloudy or foul-smelling urine, and frequent urge to urinate. Associated symptoms include nausea, vomiting, diarrhea, and decreased appetite. While some UTIs are viral, bacterial UTIs are typically treated with antibiotics. The following conventional remedies and alternatives represent prevention strategies for your consideration.

Urinary Tract Infections Side-by-Side Comparison

	Conventional Remedy	Treatment Alternative
Generic Treatment	Trimethoprim, sulfamethoxazole (TMP/SMX)	Cranberry extract
Sample Brand Name Treatment	Septra	HerbPharm Cranberry Extract

	Conventional Remedy	Treatment Alternative
How it works	Septra is an antibiotic that helps prevent bacterial colonization of the urinary tract.	Cranberry extract helps promote urinary tract health. It does not cure a urinary tract infection alone but helps prevent them from occurring by interfering with bacterial attachment to urinary tract cells.
Dosage	Dosage varies based on a child's weight or as directed by a doctor.	Take 30-40 drops per day divided into 2-3 doses.
Active Ingredients	TMP/SMX	Cranberry extract
Common Mild Side Effects	Nausea, constipation, decreased appetite, atomach pain, headache, vaginal itching or discharge, diarrhea, gas	Mild nausea
Less Common Serious Side Effects	Allergic reaction, yeast infection, numbness, fever, bloody stools	Allergic reaction

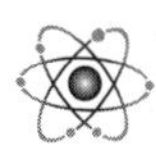

Science Says

Researchers at the Department of Pediatrics at Catholic University in Rome, Italy, studied the effectiveness of cranberry juice in the prevention of recurrent urinary tract infections. In the study, 84 girls between the ages of 3 and 14 were randomized to receive either cranberry juice, *Lactobacillus* (a friendly bacteria), or a placebo. Data from the study suggests that daily consumption of cranberry juice significantly prevents recurrence of urinary tract infections in children and was far more effective than placebo or *Lactobacillus*.

Natural Selection

In terms of natural supplements, consider D-Mannose (found naturally in cranberries, other fruits, and some plants) to prevent urinary tract infections. Like cranberry, it promotes a healthy urinary tract by interfering with bacterial attachment in the urinary tract. *Uva ursi*, known as bearberry, is an herb used to treat urinary tract infections with its antimicrobial and anti-inflammatory effects. Finally, *Echinacea*, taken in either pill or tea form, is another herb that may fight or prevent bacterial UTIs.

Spotlight On: Cranberry

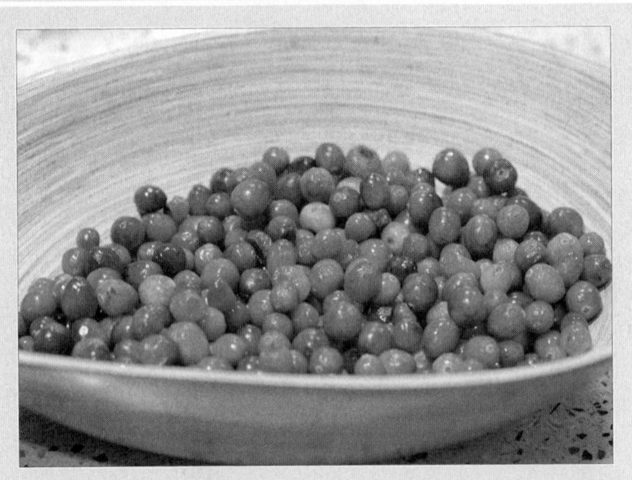

Cranberries have earned their superfood status.

We've already seen the positive effects of cranberry with respect to urinary tract infections. It turns out cranberries are considered a superfood with tremendous antioxidant properties to decrease inflammation in a host of ailments.

Cranberries contain proanthocyanidins that aid in preventing the adhesion of certain bacteria, including *E. coli,* which is commonly associated with urinary tract infections.

The anti-adhesion properties of cranberry also inhibit other bacteria, particularly those associated with gum disease and stomach ulcers.

The benefits don't stop there; recent research also shows that cranberries contain significant amounts of antioxidants and other phytonutrients that may help protect against heart disease, cancer, and other diseases. Right up there with açai berry and pomegranate, cranberry absolutely deserves to be crowned a superfood.

Of note, drinking more cranberry juice may not be particularly healthful due to higher sugar concentrations. Instead, focus on high-quality cranberry extracts either in capsule or concentrated liquid forms. Make sure your child drinks plenty of water and doesn't resist the urge to pee.

9

Dermatological Dilemmas

"Essential oils are a wonderful healing approach for children. Newborns recognize their mother by scent, not sight. Children explore the world by smelling things. As we age, a single scent can trigger a flood of memories. As you cuddle your child in your arms when sick, allowing them to smell a few drops of lemon and eucalyptus can ease their breathing and reduce their fever. As they fall asleep at night, a gentle foot or hand rub with lavender and marjoram will send them off into the sweet and gentle night with a sweet and soothing scent. Essential oils are more than a sweet smell. They calm the nerves, aid the body, and soothe the soul."

—Kamyar M. Hedayat, MD, FAAP, Medical Director, Full Spectrum Health Center for Integrative Medicine, Solana Beach, California; Founder and President, Aroma MD

Are you ready for the skinny on skin? One can't help but think of that favorite childhood joke, "Your epidermis is showing." Can you remember frantically searching your pants zipper, pockets, and other body parts only to be informed the epidermis is actually your skin? Fifteen minutes later you performed the same stunt on another unsuspecting youngster.

With skin covering our entire body, it's no wonder this chapter is chock-full of so many childhood ailments. From acne on your teenager's face to lice on your 6-year-old's scalp, we've got skin covered like sunscreen on a broiling beach day.

The good news is that many of these skin-related ailments are readily treatable, particularly with the treatment alternatives discussed for each. That's comforting for parents everywhere who see their kids scratching and itching their way through the day. So let's go from acne through warts and tackle all the dermatological dilemmas your kids face.

Acne

Acne feels like an awful practical joke on teenagers. Right at the time that appearance matters most, pimples wreak havoc on teenage confidence. Suddenly your son feels like the whole world is staring at his forehead blemishes. It can turn the most outgoing adolescent into a shy, homebound youth. It's no wonder parents are so anxious to wipe out this ailment. We all know if a kid is called "pizza face" just one time it can set him back socially for years.

Predominantly seen in teens, acne occurs when hair follicles get blocked by dirt, oil, and dead skin cells. Skin inflammation results and leads to whiteheads, blackheads, pimples, and other blemishes. While acne is most commonly found on the face, back, neck, and chest, it can spring up anywhere.

Acne can be triggered by a host of causes including stress, cosmetics, genetics (thanks, mom and dad), menstruation, and even contact with grease. For a teenager with a moderate to severe blemish breakout, the cause feels less important than trying one of the treatment alternatives discussed next.

Acne Side-by-Side Comparison

	Conventional Remedy	Treatment Alternative
Generic Treatment	Benzoyl peroxide	Tea tree oil
Sample Brand Name Treatment	Proactiv Solutions Treatment	Poofy Organics Zippy Zit Zapper

	Conventional Remedy	Treatment Alternative
How it works	Proactive treatment consists of a cleanser, toner, and lotion that exfoliate, cleanse, and repair the skin.	This treatment targets problem areas to help improve and reduce blemishes.
Dosage	Cleanser: apply dime-size amount to face and massage for 1-2 minutes and rinse 2 times daily; toner: apply dime-size amount to cotton ball and treat face 2 times daily; repairing treatment: apply pea-size amount to affected areas 2 times daily.	Apply directly to blemishes at first sign of outbreak
Active Ingredients	Benzoyl peroxide	Jojoba oil; beeswax; calendula oil; neem oil; avocado oil; essential oils of sandalwood, tea tree, galbanum, lavender, and eucalyptus; turmeric powder
Common Mild Side Effects	Dryness, swelling, irritation, redness, peeling, dark spots	None
Less Common Serious Side Effects	Allergic reaction	None

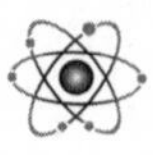

Science Says

Researchers in the Department of Dermatology at the Isfahan University of Medical Sciences in Iran studied the effectiveness of topical tea tree oil gel in treating acne. In the study, 60 patients with mild to moderate acne participated in a randomized double-blind, placebo-controlled clinical trial. Patients were followed every 15 days for a period of 6 weeks. Researchers found that patients treated with tea tree oil gel showed significant improvements in both total acne lesions and an acne severity index score compared to placebo-treated patients.

Natural Selection

If tea tree oil is not your cup of tea, consider having your teen take a zinc supplement (25 to 50 milligrams per day) to both improve skin growth and speed up blemish healing. Omega-3 fatty acids (e.g., fish or flaxseed oil) have properties to decrease skin inflammation associated with acne. Typically, 1 to 2 pills of 1,000 milligrams taken daily should be sufficient.

In Chapter 4 you learned about the benefits of honey. It's back again to help with acne, too. The hydrogen peroxide in honey has antibacterial properties. You can make a facial mask of honey and any natural exfoliant (e.g., sugar) to help remove dead skin cells and kill bacteria. Alternatively, a mask of oatmeal and water (¾:1 ratio) can help draw out oil and dirt from the skin.

Athlete's Foot

If you didn't know better, you might view athlete's foot as a compliment. You could see a sports fan saying, "Your son is such a great soccer player; he was clearly born with an athlete's foot." Then again, this book is not about compliments—rather, it focuses on ailments.

Athlete's foot, also called tinea pedis, is a contagious fungal foot infection caused by a fungus in the trichophyton family. This fungus then grows on or in the skin on any part of the feet.

✓ Good to Know

Ever wonder why it's called athlete's foot? It turns out the fungus that causes it is commonly found where athletes hang out. Pools, public showers, and locker rooms are breeding grounds for the fungus that attaches itself to barefoot athletes passing through.

The most common symptoms of athlete's foot include itching, burning, peeling, redness, blisters, or cracking skin that appears white in color. Athlete's foot is most easily prevented by wearing shoes with good air circulation, keeping feet clean and dry, and wearing flip-flops in public showers and locker rooms. However, if your child already has an outbreak, then check out these conventional remedies and treatment alternatives to help get your kid back on his feet again soon.

Athlete's Foot Side-by-Side Comparison

	Conventional Remedy	Treatment Alternative
Generic Treatment	Miconazole nitrate	Ajoene (garlic compound)
Sample Brand Name Treatment	Desenex	New Chapter Garlic Force
How it works	Desenex is an antifungal that slows the growth of fungi and helps to clear skin infections associated with athlete's foot.	New Chapter Garlic Force is a highly concentrated garlic supplement that helps treat athlete's foot. Garlic has natural antifungal properties and also provides cardiovascular support.

	Conventional Remedy	Treatment Alternative
Dosage	When affected area is clean and dry, apply Desenex 2 times per day for 2-4 weeks or as directed by a doctor.	Take 1 softgel daily with food and water or as directed by a doctor.
Active Ingredients	Miconazole	Garlic (bulb) hydroethanolic extract (min. 0.3 mg cysteine compounds), garlic (bulb) supercritical extract (min. 1.6 mg sulfur-containing compounds), parsley (seed), caraway (seed), cardamom (seed), clove (bud), fennel (seed), ginger (rhizome), peppermint (leaf)
Common Mild Side Effects	Itching, burning, rash, irritation, stinging, swelling, tenderness, flaky skin	Garlic odor (from mouth or body), heartburn
Less Common Serious Side	Allergic reaction	Allergic reaction

Science Says

Researchers at the Universidad de Oriente in Venezuela studied the effectiveness of ajoene (derived from garlic) in the short-term treatment of athlete's foot. In their study, 27 of 34 patients were completely cured of athlete's foot after 7 days of ajoene cream treatment. The remaining seven patients achieved complete cure after an additional seven days. Additionally, the 34 patients were re-checked 90 days later, and 100 percent yielded negative cultures for athlete's foot fungus.

Natural Selection

As indicted in previous section, tea tree oil is a great treatment for acne. Keep it close by for athlete's foot, too. Dispense several drops on a cotton ball and apply topically to the affected area one or two times per day. The tea tree oil acts like an antiseptic to help eliminate the fungus. You can also apply cornstarch to your child's feet to keep the infected area dry while helping soothe associated irritation. Finally, soaking your child's feet in a mixture of equal parts warm water and apple cider vinegar will relieve itching, redness, and athlete's foot inflammation.

Chicken Pox

Poor chickens! Don't they have enough to worry about without an errant link to a contagious viral infection? Come to think of it, dogs also have to overcome the negative connotation associated with "sick as a dog." And don't get me started on "pigeon-toed"!

Chicken pox is caused by a virus called varicella-zoster and results in red, itchy, raised bumps that can cover any part of your child's skin. These red blisters usually develop within two days of contact with the virus.

✓ Good to Know

So why are chickens linked to the pox? Some folks believe the small spots look like something a chicken beak could cause from incessant pecking. Another common theory stems from the supposed resemblance of chicken pox spots to chickpeas once the rash blisters.

Beyond the red, raised bumps, other chicken pox symptoms include sore throat, fever, headache, and an upset stomach. Children are generally exposed to chicken pox by other infected kids. It can also develop in adults who have not been exposed to the virus as a child. If your child is already itching, scratching, and blaming chickens, you'll want to review these treatment alternatives closely.

Chicken Pox Side-by-Side Comparison

	Conventional Remedy	Treatment Alternative
Generic Treatment	Diphenhydramine	Oatmeal
Sample Brand Name Treatment	Benadryl (Children's Allergy Liquid)	Aveeno Baby Soothing Bath Treatment
How it works	Benadryl Children's Allergy Liquid is an antihistamine that helps provide relief from the symptoms associated with chicken pox.	When added to a bath, Aveeno Baby Soothing Bath Treatment provides relief from symptoms of chicken pox while also moisturizing the skin.
Dosage	Children ages 6 and up: take 5-10mL every 4-6 hours. Do not exceed 6 doses in 24 hours.	Sprinkle powder under faucet in a bathtub of warm water. Use once per day in a 15-20 minute bath or as directed by a doctor.
Active Ingredients	Diphenhydramine HCl 12.5mg	Colloidal oatmeal
Common Mild Side Effects	Drowsiness, weakness, excitability, dry mouth or nose, constipation, diarrhea, headache, nausea, vomiting, decreased appetite	None
Less Common Serious Side Effects	Allergic reaction, irregular heartbeat, difficulty urinating or inability to urinate, chills, fever, dizziness, seizure, severe drowsiness, tremor, changes in vision, unexplained bruising or bleeding	Allergic reaction

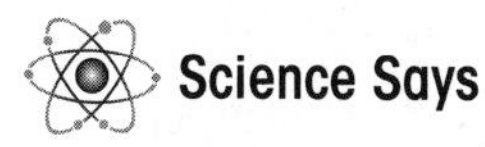

Science Says

The Department of Dermatology at Royal London Hospital in the UK reviewed the mechanism of action and clinical benefits of colloidal oatmeal in dermatologic practice. It turns out that avenanthramides, components of whole oat grain, give oatmeal its anti-inflammatory and antihistaminic properties. Researchers concluded that "topical formulations of natural colloidal oatmeal should be considered an important component of therapy" for itchy skin conditions.

Natural Selection

If you want to save the oatmeal for breakfast tomorrow, instead consider spreading honey over areas affected by chicken pox. Ignore the sticky factor and instead appreciate the itching relief for your little one. Soaking in a warm bath with two to three tablespoons of baking soda may help the blisters heal more quickly. You can also add a teaspoon of powdered ginger to the bath as an alternative to the baking soda. Finally, apple cider vinegar poured on a cotton ball and applied to affected areas will relieve itching.

Eczema

How many words can you think of that start with the letters *ecz*? If you only thought of one, you're ready for the spelling bee. You're also ready to learn about eczema.

A skin condition that mainly affects babies and toddlers, eczema can cause itchiness and raised, bumpy, scaly rashes on the skin. Common symptoms include visible irritation and inflammation of the skin, dry or scaly skin, oozing blisters, and red patches. These irritations are typically seen on the face, neck, hands, and feet.

While eczema may be hereditary, it can also be caused by a number of environmental factors. These include exposure to extreme temperatures, allergies, unusual fabrics, perfumes and dyes, or exposure to topical irritants.

If you're done trying to spell eczema and are ready to learn the remedy choices available, keep reading for a side-by-side comparison of hydrocortisone and licorice gel.

Eczema Side-by-Side Comparison

	Conventional Remedy	Treatment Alternative
Generic Treatment	Hydrocortisone	Licorice gel
Sample Brand Name Treatment	Cortaid 1%	Atopiclair
How it works	Cortaid is an anti-inflammatory steroid applied topically that helps relieve redness, irritation, itching, inflammation, and rashes on a temporary basis.	Atopiclair provides necessary moisture and soothes the skin while also helping to prevent future eczema outbreaks. It is nonsteroidal.
Dosage	Apply to skin 1-4 times per day to the affected area after cleaning it. Use just enough to cover the affected area. Do not use on children prior to consulting a doctor.	Children ages 6 mo. and older: apply 2-3 times per day or as needed on the affected area. Consult a doctor before use.
Active Ingredients	Hydrocortisone	Glycyrrhetinic acid, hyaluronic acid

	Conventional Remedy	Treatment Alternative
Common Mild Side Effects	Burning sensation, itching, peeling of the skin, redness, dryness, changes in skin tone, cracked skin, blisters	Mild burning, stinging, redness
Less Common Serious Side Effects	Allergic reaction, irregular heartbeat, fatigue, blurred vision, skin infection, unexplained weight gain, insomnia	Allergic reaction

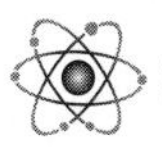

Science Says

Researchers at the Department of Pharmaceutics at Mazandaran University in Iran studied the treatment of atopic dermatitis (eczema) with licorice gel. Two licorice gel formulations (1 and 2 percent) were studied in double-blind clinical trials with 60 patients. The 2 percent solution seemed most effective in reducing itching over a period of two weeks, although both preparations were effective in treating atopic dermatitis.

Natural Selection

Primrose oil can help reduce inflammation, itching, and redness associated with eczema. Chamomile or calendula cream can also reduce inflammation when used topically as an eczema treatment. Aloe vera or grapefruit seed extract can also provide similar soothing relief. Finally, eczema outbreaks can be reduced and outbreak recoveries sped up through probiotics to support a healthy immune system.

Head Lice

Do you remember head lice check day in school when you were young? You'd be working feverishly on multiplication tables when an intercom announcement signaled your turn to hike to the nurse's office. There a friendly lady in white would meticulously comb through your hair looking for nits. Nervous principals everywhere wanted to prevent school-wide lice breakouts.

Lice are tiny insects that find comfort and refuge on the scalp of unsuspecting people everywhere. Human-to-human contact or sharing brushes, combs, and clothing can transmit lice. Head lice can be found in any part of the hair or scalp but are most commonly seen in the hair shaft closest to the scalp surface.

Lice symptoms include itchy scalp, visible lice or eggs (nits), a tickling sensation on the head, or scalp scabs caused by itching. While head lice are not life-threatening, they certainly wreak havoc on families, and these conventional remedies and treatment alternatives can speed the recovery process considerably.

Head Lice Side-by-Side Comparison

	Conventional Remedy	Treatment Alternative
Generic Treatment	Permethrin	Dimethicone
Sample Brand Name Treatment	Nix	LiceMD
How it works	Nix treats head lice by killing adult lice and nits, which are their eggs.	LiceMD does not contain pesticides and is an odorless treatment to get rid of lice and nits.

	Conventional Remedy	Treatment Alternative
Dosage	Children ages 2 months and older: after shampooing, place Nix so that it covers hair and scalp. Leave on for 10 minutes, rinse with warm water, towel dry hair and comb to remove tangles; remove lice and nits with comb provided.	Apply LiceMD to dry hair and leave on for 10 minutes before sectioning and combing hair to remove lice and nits. Then rinse hair with shampoo and warm water. Be sure to use a nit comb, which is extremely fine toothed, to catch the tiny nits in the comb.
Active Ingredients	Permethrin 280mg	Dimethicone
Common Mild Side Effects	Mild burning, itching, swelling, redness, stinging, tingling	None
Less Common Serious Side Effects	Allergic reaction, seizures	None

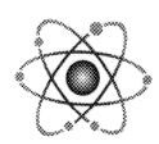

Science Says

Scientists at the Department of Community Health at the Federal University of Ceara in Brazil compared permethrin and dimethicone in the treatment of head lice. In the study, 145 children, ages 5 to 15 years, were treated twice with either dimethicone or permethrin over a nine-day period. After two days, 95 percent of children treated with dimethicone were cured versus 67 percent of those treated with permethrin. Resistance to permethrin and other lice neurotoxins has been increasing over time; however, scientists hypothesized that the development of resistance is highly unlikely for dimethicone since it interrupts lice's oxygen supply to the central nervous system.

Natural Selection

Tea tree oil is back again as the MVP of this chapter. Adding 10 drops to 2 ounces of olive oil can help eliminate lice and nits when applied to the scalp and hair and combed through. The solution should be rinsed out of the hair after three to four hours. Both lavender oil and coconut oil are also effective. Lavender oil contains terpenoids, a natural chemical that helps repel lice. Coconut oil can be applied to the scalp and covered with a shower cap for several hours. Rinse and comb afterward to wash out the lice and nits.

Alternatively, Aviva Romm, MD, suggests a mixture of ⅓ cup of olive oil (for the average sized head) and 10 drops of essential oil of thyme. Apply liberally to the scalp and cover the head with a plastic shower cap (not plastic bags!). Leave on for 30 minutes, shampoo well, and repeat in one week.

Impetigo

Have you ever heard of *Staphylococcus aureus* or *Streptococcus pyogenes*? Chances are these words seem nonsensical to you, like something out of Dr. Seuss's catalog—unless, of course, your son or daughter suffers from impetigo. These happen to be the two bacteria most responsible for this skin infection.

Impetigo results in rashes and blisters that can appear on the face, neck, hands, arms, and legs. The most common symptoms are oozing blisters, red spots, itchiness, crusty skin, and ruptured sores. Kids typically contract impetigo when the bacteria infiltrate an open wound from a cut, bite, or other injury.

Impetigo comes in two types. The first is bullous impetigo, which causes blisters filled with fluid. The second type of impetigo is non-bullous, which causes crusty lesions on the skin. Whichever type your child may have contracted, you'll want to check out the treatment options covered here.

Impetigo Side-by-Side Comparison

	Conventional Remedy	Treatment Alternative
Generic Treatment	Mupirocin	Manuka honey
Sample Brand Name Treatment	Bactroban	HNZ Bio Active Manuka Honey
How it works	Bactroban is a topical ointment that helps treat skin infections such as impetigo by preventing bacterial growth.	HNZ Bio Active Manuka Honey contains unique antibacterial qualities that help cure infectious conditions such as impetigo.
Dosage	Children ages 2 months and older: apply ointment to affected areas up to 3 times per day or as directed by a doctor. Clean and dry areas prior to application.	After cleaning and drying the area, apply Manuka honey to areas affected by impetigo.
Active Ingredients	Mupirocin	Pure manuka floral honey
Common Mild Side Effects	Dry skin, burning irritation, redness, itching, rash, stinging, swelling, pain, nausea, headache	Mild skin irritation
Less Common Serious Side Effects	Allergic reaction, severe itching, severe skin irritation	None (Botulism is listed, but that is only a risk if Manuka Honey is ingested by infants under 1 year).

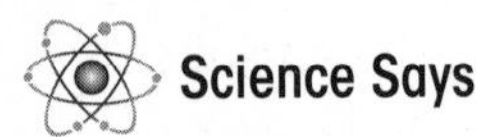

Science Says

The Department of Biological Sciences at the University of Waikato in New Zealand studied seven major wound-infecting bacteria species to compare their sensitivity to both manuka honey (non-peroxide antibacterial activity) and another honey with hydrogen peroxide–based antibacterial activity. Researchers discovered that manuka honey at a concentration of 1.8 percent completely inhibited the growth of *Staphylococcus aureus* during incubation for eight hours.

Natural Selection

Get your oils out if you want to help treat your child's impetigo. Oil of oregano has natural antibiotic properties that help clear impetigo-associated bacteria. Cinnamon oil, when applied topically one or two times per day also treats impetiginized wounds. Myrrh oil has both antibacterial and anti-inflammatory qualities to help relieve and heal impetigo outbreaks. When applying essential oils, remember they are typically mixed with a carrier oil like olive oil. Finally, coconut oil can help dry the impetigo sores and speed the healing process.

Minor Skin Infections

When your little one is crying in pain, the word *minor* never enters your vocabulary. Every scratch, itch, and wince can make a parent nervous. However, this section is all about the word *minor*, as in minor skin infections.

Bacteria, fungi, and viruses share the blame for minor skin infections. Any of the three can enter the skin through a scrape, cut, or similar wound or skin condition. Allergies or exposure to irritants can also lead to minor skin infections. Many common ailments also lead to minor skin infections including impetigo, bug bites, and chicken pox—all of which are covered in this book.

Regardless of how the skin infection is contracted, your little one will likely show one or more symptoms, including visible redness, rash, and blisters. As these symptoms emerge, you'll want to check out the conventional remedies and treatment alternatives available to prevent something minor from turning into something major.

Minor Skin Infections Side-by-Side Comparison

	Conventional Remedy	Treatment Alternative
Generic Treatment	Benzalkonium chloride, lidocaine HCl	Vitamin E
Sample Brand Name Treatment	Bactine	Jason 45000IU Vitamin E Pure Beauty Oil
How it works	Bactine helps provide relief of pain associated with minor skin infections by cleansing the area and providing protection from infection.	Jason 45000IU Vitamin E Pure Beauty Oil helps to reduce inflammation and protect the skin while also leaving it nourished and moisturized. It is an antioxidant that promotes skin regeneration.
Dosage	Children under 2 years of age: consult a doctor before use; children ages 2 years and older: clean affected area and apply topically 1-3 times per day.	After cleaning skin, apply topically as needed to affected areas.
Active Ingredients	Benzalkonium Cl 0.13% w/w, lidocaine HCl 2.5% w/w	Vitamin E
Common Mild Side Effects	Redness, swelling, mild irritation, numbness at application site	None

	Conventional Remedy	Treatment Alternative
Less Common Serious Side Effects	Allergic reaction, choking, dizziness, impaired thought process, lightheadedness, fever, irregular heartbeat, seizure, swelling of the throat, changes in vision, ringing in the ears	None

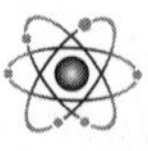

Science Says

Scientists at the Department of Surgical Sciences at the University of Verona in Italy studied the effects of topical vitamin E on minor skin ailments in children. In the study, vitamin E was used 3 times daily for 15 days prior to surgery and then twice daily for 30 days post-surgery. Results showed that 96 percent of patients (or their parents) considered cosmetic results to be very good. Zero patients endured any wound infections after vitamin E treatment. In contrast, only 78 percent of the control group who received a placebo viewed cosmetic results as very good.

Natural Selection

Hydrogen peroxide can be used to disinfect and cleanse a minor skin infection. Simply pour a small amount directly on the infection. Alternatively, your child can soak in a warm bath with ⅓ to ½ bottle of hydrogen peroxide added. In lieu of hydrogen peroxide, thyme oil can be applied topically to the skin to both provide relief and hasten the healing process. Additionally, peppermint oil and clove oil are useful in treating minor infections of the skin. Peppermint oil soothes the skin and reduces inflammation while clove oil acts as a skin disinfectant. And, once again, tea tree oil may be a good option in cases of minor skin infections (as mentioned previously, use only a few drops of each essential oil mixed with a teaspoon of carrier oil (like olive oil) before applying to the skin).

Molluscum

Don't be confused in this section. Molluscum is not the specialty of the day at an upscale seafood restaurant; you're thinking of mollusks—common seafood favorites like clams, oysters, scallops, and mussels.

Molluscum has nothing to do with seafood. It's actually a contagious skin virus in the pox family that causes raised bumps on the skin. The official name is molluscum contagiosum, and this virus is spread through contact with any skin or items already infected with the virus.

The defining characteristic of this ailment is bumps that are hard and either pink or white in color. The bumps may closely match your child's skin color. These bumps are typically the size of a freckle and most commonly appear on the face, neck, arms, and hands. They can be confused with warts.

Without treatment, these bumps can last as long as 6 to 12 months. If you're looking for a quicker fix, one of the remedies covered here could be your best bet.

Molluscum Side-by-Side Comparison

	Conventional Remedy	Treatment Alternative
Generic Treatment	Cryotherapy	Australian lemon myrtle
Sample Brand Name Treatment	Liquid nitrogen	Tea Tree Therapy Lemon Myrtle 100% Essential Oil
How it works	Cryotherapy uses liquid nitrogen to freeze off bumps caused by the molluscum virus. Temperatures of -320°F are employed for this purpose.	Lemon myrtle oil is an antibacterial that helps treat skin issues such as bumps caused by the molluscum virus

	Conventional Remedy	Treatment Alternative
Dosage	Applied directly to the bumps or lesions, the course of treatment is performed by and determined by a doctor.	Add 2 drops of lemon myrtle oil to a tsp of carrier oil such as vegetable oil and massage onto skin where bumps appear. Apply to bump sites with a cotton ball or swab 1-3 times daily to help diminish molluscum bumps.
Active Ingredients	Liquid nitrogen	Pure lemon myrtle oil
Common Mild Side Effects	Inflammation at the treatment site, blistering, bleeding, headache, hair loss, changes in pigmentation	Skin irritation
Less Common Serious Side Effects	Scarring, fainting, heavy bleeding, burns, fever, chills, nerve damage	Allergic reaction

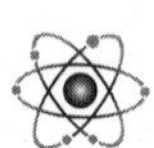

Science Says

The Center for Biomedical Research in Boise, Idaho, conducted research on Australian lemon myrtle in the treatment of molluscum contagiosum in children. Thirty-one children with a mean age of 4½ were treated with either a once-daily topical application of a 10 percent solution of Australian lemon myrtle or simply olive oil. After 21 days, 9 of the 16 children treated with lemon myrtle oil showed a 90 percent or greater reduction in the number of lesions. Those treated with olive oil showed no improvement.

Natural Selection

ZymaDerm is a homeopathic treatment for molluscum. Safe for ages 9 months and older, it is applied topically to molluscum bumps twice daily for 30 days. The homeopathic remedy *Thuja occidentalis* can speed up the healing process for molluscum. Finally, adding ⅓ to ½ cup of apple cider vinegar to a warm bath for your child and soaking for 15-20 minutes can help heal molluscum bumps.

Psoriasis

Growth and *acceleration* are usually promising terms associated with a child's development. This is not the case when it comes to psoriasis. For kids suffering from this ailment, the growth of skin cells is accelerated, resulting in a buildup of dead skin cells on the skin's surface.

While psoriasis is a chronic condition thought to be genetic, it is not believed to be contagious. The most common symptoms include patches of red, dry skin that can appear anywhere on the body. These patches may also be white or silver in appearance. Beyond the patches, additional symptoms include joint pain, discolored or thickened nails, and moderate to severe dandruff.

✓ Good to Know

Psoriasis is most commonly found in people ages 15 to 35. However, 10 to 15 percent of people with psoriasis show symptoms before the age of 10. In total, approximately 20,000 children under the age of 10 are diagnosed with psoriasis annually in the United States. It is often confused with eczema.

Psoriasis is believed to initiate through immune system flare-ups from a number of causes. These include stress, dry skin, skin wounds, and viral or bacterial illnesses. The treatment options, including conventional and alternative, are covered here.

Psoriasis Side-by-Side Comparison

	Conventional Remedy	Treatment Alternative
Generic Treatment	Betamethasone	Topical vitamin D (calcipotriene)
Sample Brand Name Treatment	Valisone	Dovonex ointment
How it works	Applied topically, Valisone helps to treat symptoms of psoriasis like redness, itching, pain, dryness, and inflammation of the skin.	Dovonex is synthetic vitamin D that helps to treat existing patches of skin that are red, inflamed, or itchy due to psoriasis.
Dosage	Use only as directed by a doctor, as children are more sensitive to Valisone than adults.	Consult doctor before use in children. Typical dosage of topical treatment: 2 times per day to affected areas; avoid contact with eyes and face.
Active Ingredients	Betamethasone (steroid)	Calcipotriene Ingredients
Common Mild Side Effects	Itching, burning, skin dryness or cracking, changes in pigmentation, blistering, peeling	Skin irritation, rash, itching, inflammation, worsened psoriasis, redness, dryness, burning
Less Common Serious Side Effects	Allergic reaction, skin infection, blurred vision, irregular heartbeat, insomnia, weight gain, fatigue, changes in behavior	Allergic reaction, severe burning or swelling, changes in pigmentation

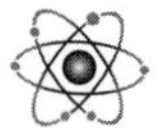

Science Says

Researchers in the Department of Dermatology at Radboud University Nijmegan Medical Center in the Netherlands conducted a systematic review of treatments for childhood psoriasis. In total, scientists examined 64 completed studies from previous trials. Upon review, calcipotriene was noted to be the most effective topical treatment for psoriasis.

Natural Selection

Phototherapy treatments, performed by a doctor, can help treat psoriasis flare-ups by slowing the growth of skin cells through exposure to ultraviolet light. To ease the itching associated with psoriasis, consider a bath with one cup of baking soda or the liberal application of aloe to psoriasis patches.

Ringworm

Digging for worms on a rainy day is a favorite childhood pastime. The same is not true for ringworm. While not actually a worm of any type, this fungal skin infection is contagious and typically contracted through skin contact with another infected person.

Ring-shaped red skin is the calling card for ringworm; this unique shape differentiates it from other skin-related ailments covered in this book. The ring-shaped discoloration may appear anywhere throughout the body including the arms, hands, legs, feet, and scalp. The skin may also appear itchy and scaly, especially around the edges. Ringworm can also spread to the nails, causing discoloration and possible nail breakage. It can even cause localized hair loss when spread to the scalp.

If you're ready to see your child's focus back on digging for worms, then you'll want to tackle ringworm with one of the treatment alternatives covered in this section.

Ringworm Side-by-Side Comparison

	Conventional Remedy	Treatment Alternative
Generic Treatment	Fluconazole	Tea tree oil
Sample Brand Name Treatment	Diflucan	Aroma MD Tea Tree Oil
How it works	Diflucan is an antibiotic that helps treat fungal infections such as ringworm.	Tea tree oil helps to dry out and kill the ringworm fungus.
Dosage	Use only as directed by a doctor; common dosage in children is 3mg taken orally once per day for 1-2 weeks.	Apply 1-2 drops of tea tree oil to a cotton swab and apply to area affected by ringworm up to 3 times per day for up to 4 weeks.
Active Ingredients	Fluconazole	Tea tree oil
Common Mild Side Effects	Diarrhea, dizziness, upset stomach, headache, changes in pigmentation, unusual taste or changes in perception of food	Skin irritation or sensitivity, dryness, itching, redness, stinging
Less Common Serious Side Effects	Allergic reaction, extreme fatigue, lethargy, decreased appetite, pain in the upper right part of the stomach, jaundice, seizure, pale stools, dark urine, bruising	Allergic reaction, severe burning or swelling

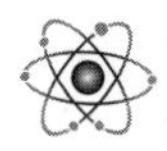

Science Says

At the Universita Politecnica delle Marche in Ancona, Italy, researchers investigated the susceptibility of fungi to both conventional and alternative antifungal agents. They discovered tea tree oil compounds to be as effective as fluconazole (antifungal medication) in the treatment of fungi that cause tinea (ringworm).

Natural Selection

If tea tree oil doesn't improve the condition, consider one of these treatment alternatives. Note that all of these may take some time to work, so repeat three times per day for 2-4 weeks as needed.

- Mix a clove of crushed garlic with olive oil and honey and apply to the affected area. Cover with a bandage for two hours before washing.
- Using a carrier oil (like olive oil), add 3-5 drops of lavender oil or lemongrass oil and massage into affected ringworm areas to relieve inflammation and itchiness.
- Apply coconut oil topically to the affected area to help treat ringworm.

Warts

They say you've got to love your soulmate warts and all. However, when it comes to your kids, why not eliminate warts from the equation when truly effective treatment options exist?

A wart is a small growth on the skin caused by the human papillomavirus (HPV). This virus finds its way into your child's skin through any type of break in the skin such as a wound or open sore.

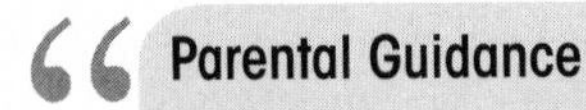

Parental Guidance

"One of my daughters showed me a cluster of three or four tiny bumps on the bottom of her foot. The podiatrist confirmed they were warts. Remembering the painful treatment I received for a wart as a child, I feared the worst for my daughter. But surprisingly, the podiatrist suggested a much easier and pain-free suggestion. Since we had caught the warts early, all we had to do was keep them covered with duct tape—yes, duct tape!—for approximately six weeks. The duct tape would smother and eventually kill the virus. Sure enough, six weeks later the podiatrist confirmed the warts were gone! He stressed that catching them early was key. An older, deeper wart is less likely to respond to this treatment."

—Alyssa, mother to 9-year-old twin daughters Samantha and Rebecca

The biggest indicator of warts is the presence of small growths that are typically round or oval in shape, and they are most commonly seen on the hands, feet, or face. Warts can be smooth or rough in texture—or even completely flat. They may appear to be pink, brown, grayish-white, or even flesh-colored.

In total, there are six different types of warts:

1. Common warts, which appear most frequently on the hands.
2. Filiform warts, which usually show up on the face.
3. Flat warts, which may appear on the face, neck, or hands.
4. Periungal warts, which show up on or around the toenails or fingernails.
5. Plantar warts, which are usually seen on the feet.
6. Genital warts, which, as their name indicates, show up in the genital area.

Regardless of the type of wart, you'll want to understand the treatment options for your child. If the wart is in the facial region, you may want to skip the duct tape recommendation and scan ahead to the natural selection of treatment alternatives covered at the end of this section. Your child will thank you for not making them leave the house with duct tape stuck to their face.

Warts Side-by-Side Comparison

	Conventional Remedy	Treatment Alternative
Generic Treatment	Salicylic acid	Duct tape
Sample Brand Name Treatment	Compound W (Fast Acting Gel)	Tyco
How it works	Applied topically, Compound W helps shed the skin cells that are affected by warts and also helps prevent the virus from spreading to other areas.	Duct type prompts an immune response that gradually kills the HPV virus and eventually eliminates the presence of warts.
Dosage	Wash affected area in warm water for 5 minutes, dry thoroughly and apply enough gel to cover wart; let dry and repeat 1-2 times per day as needed for up to 12 weeks. Recommended only for children ages 4 and older.	Apply enough duct tape to completely cover the wart and leave firmly in place for 6 days; remove tape and soak skin before exfoliating the site to remove dead skin cells. Repeat as needed until wart is gone.
Active Ingredients	Salicylic acid	Polyethylene, adhesive, cloth
Common Mild Side Effects	Minor redness or skin irritation, dry skin	Skin irritation

	Conventional Remedy	Treatment Alternative
Less Common Serious Side Effects	Allergic reaction, severe skin irritation, severe burning sensation	Allergic reaction

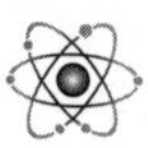

Science Says

At the Children's Hospital Medical Center in Cincinnati, Ohio, researchers compared the effectiveness of duct tape versus cryotherapy in treating the common wart. In total, 61 patients, ages 3 to 22, were included in the study. Half the trial participants received cryotherapy (liquid nitrogen) applied to each wart for 10 seconds every two weeks for a maximum of six treatments. The other half of participants wore duct tape over the warts for a period of two months. At the conclusion of the study, 85 percent of those treated with duct tape versus 60 percent of those treated with cryotherapy had complete resolution of their warts.

Natural Selection

Curious George would be thrilled to find out banana peels are another effective treatment for warts. Simply cover the wart with a piece of banana peel—the potassium found inside helps kill the virus associated with warts.

If the wart is on a visible part of the body when fully clothed, then banana peels and duct tape may not fly with your child. Instead consider the milky, juicy substance that comes from a milkweed plant. When applied topically to a wart and covered, it can diminish the wart. Aloe vera can also reduce the presence of warts when applied directly to the wart and covered.

Spotlight On: Essential Oils

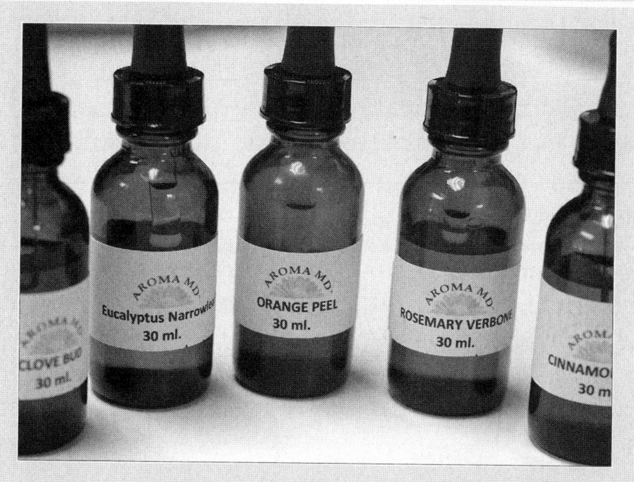

A variety of plant-based essential oils.

Essential oils are volatile liquids distilled from leaves, flowers, roots, stems, or flowers of a plant. Essential oils are highly concentrated and contain the true essence of the plant from which they are derived. Each oil has multiple chemical constituents with powerful healing potential.

The antimicrobial properties of essential oils have been known for many centuries in cultures throughout the world. Only in the last 20 to 25 years have a large number of essential oils been scientifically investigated for their antibacterial and antifungal qualities. The Institute of General Food Chemistry in Lodz, Poland, conducted one such comprehensive study. Overall, researchers found that essential oils of spices and herbs— particularly thyme, origanum, mint, cinnamon, salvia, and clove—contained the strongest antimicrobial properties.

Essential oils can serve numerous purposes in a healthy lifestyle for your child. They've appeared throughout this book as treatment alternatives, particularly in the natural selection sections at the end of each ailment covered.

Beyond just helping cure and treat childhood ailments, essential oils have found their way into aromatherapy, massage therapy, personal care, nutritional supplements, and even household cleaners.

Of course, it's important to remember that essential oils are typically highly concentrated and should be kept stored far away from the grasp of children. However, when used appropriately, essential oils have shown value across a wide spectrum of ailments including wounds, colds, and fevers. That adds to the meaning behind *essential* in their name!

10

First Aid for Bumps, Burns, Bruises, and Bites

"The FDA declared its intent to regulate sunscreens back in 1978. The rules are still in bureaucratic limbo. While regulators delay, sunscreen makers can sell products that overstate sun protection and underperform in the real world. The Environmental Working Group (EWG) continues to pressure the FDA to issue enforceable rules for sunscreen products. In the meantime, the EWG publishes the annual Sunscreen Guide rating more than 1,700 products on the market."

—Ken Cook, President and Co-founder of the Environmental Working Group (www.ewg.org)

Sometimes a kiss is all your child needs in order to soothe a bump, burn, bruise, or bite. Many a parent has watched pain and suffering melt away from a simple kiss placed in just the right spot. This is particularly effective for babies and toddlers. Unfortunately, with age comes the reality that your kid may want something more than a smooch to make the pain go away. Further, sometimes babies and toddlers need more than your lips to ease the pain.

This chapter is all about times when a kiss just won't suffice. We'll be talking about those pesky bugs and insects that sting and bite. We'll be covering sprains, cuts, scrapes, and bruises from falls and other accidents. Aloe vera will come up repeatedly as we treat burns from the sun and other causes. This chapter will even take you through the best natural treatments for nosebleeds, poison ivy, hives, and even dehydration.

By all means, try the kiss first. It's the best natural remedy around. However, if you need a little something more in the first aid department, then check out the treatment alternatives discussed here.

Bee Stings

How could something as delicious as honey come from an insect as pesky as a bee? When you're pouring honey into tea or enjoying delicious apples dipped in honey, a bee sting is the furthest thing from your mind. Sometimes you've got to take the good with the bad—if honey is here to stay, then the bee sting is too!

When a bee stings, it injects venom into the sting site, thereby affecting the body's immune system and skin near the sting. The typical bee sting leads to pain, redness, itching, and swelling around the sting site. For those with bee sting allergies, the reaction is more severe and can include difficulty breathing, hives, dizziness, nausea, and vomiting. In rare allergic reactions, loss of consciousness can even ensue. Severe allergic reactions of this type are called anaphylaxis and can be fatal if immediate medical attention is not sought.

✓ Good to Know

Did you know that nearly two million Americans are severely allergic to bee stings? It's one thing to endure the pain of a sting, it's quite another to have an allergic reaction. If your child is severely allergic to bee stings, you should always have an epinephrine auto-injector pen with you. It could be a lifesaver.

You'll identify stings on your child mainly through seeing a raised red spot with a red or white mark in the center of the sting site. The stinging or pinching sensation is usually instantaneous, so your child's shriek is likely another identifier. While symptoms will often heal within one to three days (or up to a week in rare cases), these treatment alternatives can speed up the healing process and get your child back to appreciating the joys of honey again.

Bee Stings Side-by-Side Comparison

	Conventional Remedy	Treatment Alternative
Generic Treatment	Ibuprofen	Apis Mellifica
Sample Brand Name Treatment	Children's Motrin	Boiron Apis Mellifica
How it works	Children's Motrin temporarily relieves aches and pains, such as those associated with a bee sting, for up to 8 hours.	Boiron Apis Mellifica 30C helps relieve symptoms of bee stings such as swelling.
Dosage	Under 2 years old: ask a doctor; 24-35 lbs/2-3 years: 1 tsp; 36-47 lbs/4-5 years: 1.5 tsp; 48-59 lbs/6-8 years: 2 tsp; 60-71 lbs/9-10 years: 2.5 tsp; 72-95 lbs/11 years: 3 tsp. Repeat as needed every 6-8 hours. Do not exceed 4 doses per day.	Dissolve 5 tablets by mouth 3 times per day or as directed by a doctor until symptoms subside.
Active Ingredients	Ibuprofen	Apis Mellifica 30C HPUS
Common Mild Side Effects	Drowsiness, dizziness, nausea, vomiting, diarrhea, constipation, headache, upset stomach	None

	Conventional Remedy	Treatment Alternative
Less Common Serious Side Effects	Allergic reaction, unexplained bruises or bleeding, changes in mood, hearing or vision impairment, stiffness, unusual weight gain, jaundice, dark urine, chest pain, fainting, irregular heartbeat, extreme fatigue or dizziness, dark vomit	None

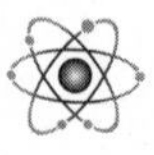

Science Says

Homeopathic Apis theoretically works in ways akin to sublingual immunotherapy (allergen solution given under the tongue to reduce sensitivity to allergens) as "like cures like." While there is no specific study on homeopathic Apis, researchers at Johns Hopkins Asthma and Allergy Center in Baltimore, Maryland, studied the outcomes of insect sting allergies in children with and without venom immunotherapy (using a very weakened form of venom). Studies found that bee venom immunotherapy significantly reduced allergic reactions to stings.

Natural Selection

Ice can help instantaneously numb the pain at the site of a sting. Simply apply the ice for 15 minutes, remove for 45 minutes, and repeat as necessary. You can even wrap the ice in a towel if it's too cold for your child. Also, a homemade paste of baking soda and water can be applied to the sting site to reduce pain and swelling. A clove of garlic can also help reduce pain and swelling symptoms. Cut the clove of garlic in half and apply the inner part of the clove directly to the sting site.

Bruises

If you've ever suffered a bruised ego, first aid was not top of mind. A little soul-searching and confidence-boosting likely soothed you back to good. Physical bruises are anything but emotional, and that's what this section is all about.

When capillaries break under the skin's surface, a bruise is the usual result. That traditional black and blue coloring of the skin is the telltale sign of a bruise and can be attributed to blood flowing under the skin from the broken capillaries.

Physical trauma is most often to blame for a bruise. This can come from falling, banging, hitting, or any other type of physical contact that doesn't result in skin breakage. Also referred to as a contusion, bruises are temporary and can last from a few days to a few weeks depending on the severity of the injury.

Your child's skin will often change colors during the healing process. The initial black and blue coloring may shift to yellow, purple, or brown throughout the healing time. The bruise site may feel tender to the touch for him as the tissue beneath the skin is tender from the bruise. As he copes with the bruise, the following treatment alternatives can provide relief and expedite the healing process.

Bruises Side-by-Side Comparison

	Conventional Remedy	Treatment Alternative
Generic Treatment	Acetaminophen	*Arnica montana*
Sample Brand Name Treatment	Children's Tylenol Liquid Suspension	Hyland's Bumps and Bruises (Tablets)

	Conventional Remedy	Treatment Alternative
How it works	Children's Tylenol helps temporarily relieve pain caused by bruising.	Hyland's Bumps and Bruises is a natural treatment using homeopathic ingredients to provide first aid and pain relief for injuries such as bruises.
Dosage	Under 24 lbs/under 2 years: consult doctor; 24-35 lbs/2-3 years: 1 tsp or 5mL; 36-47 lbs/4-5 years: 1.5 tsp or 7.5mL; 48-59 lbs/6-8 years: 2 tsp or 10mL, 60-71 lbs/9-10 years: 2.5 tsp or 12.5mL, 72-95 lbs/11 years: 3 tsp or 15mL; repeat dose every 4 hours as needed; do not exceed doses in 24 hours	Take 3-4 dissolvable tablets immediately after injury and every 15 minutes as needed to relieve pain. Tablets may also be dissolved in water and sipped. Dosage is for children ages 1 year and older.
Active Ingredients	Acetaminophen	*Arnica Montana* 6X HPUS, *Hypericum perforatum* 6X HPUS, *Bellis perennis* 6X HPUS, *Ruta graveolens* 6X HPUS
Common Mild Side Effects	Constipation, diarrhea, drowsiness, trouble sleeping	None
Less Common Serious Side Effects	Allergic reaction, liver damage, stomach pain, dizziness, changes in vision, irregular heartbeat, difficulty urinating	None

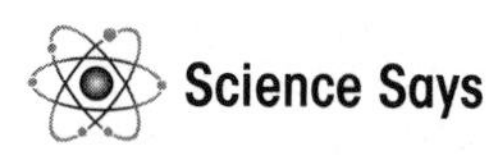

Science Says

Scientists at the Department of Dermatology at the Northwestern University Feinberg School of Medicine in Chicago, Illinois, studied the effectiveness of arnica in treating bruises. In the study, half of participants had bruises treated with a 20 percent arnica solution while the other half received a placebo. Photos of the bruises were taken on day one and after two weeks for comparison. Results showed bruising healed significantly faster for those patients treated with the 20 percent arnica solution.

Natural Selection

Consider bromelain, a natural enzyme with anti-inflammatory properties, to help minimize bruising. It's naturally found in pineapple and can be taken as a supplement, too. Vitamin C also helps as it naturally strengthens blood vessels, thereby protecting the body from injury-associated bruises. In fact, vitamin C deficiencies can lead to easier bruising in kids. Finally, to help with pain and swelling after bruising, consider ice or a cold compress on the spot of the bruise.

Burns

What is it about toddler fingers that they're programmed to instinctively reach for ovens, candles, and stovetops? That flame is so enticing for little fingers, yet touching it can be disastrous. It's no wonder parents try so hard to train kids to stay away from fire from babyhood on.

A burn is classified as a flesh injury typically caused by exposure or contact with heat, chemicals, light, fire, or electricity. Burns are classified into three categories based on severity and depth of the burn:

- First-degree burns: affecting the epidermis or outermost layer of the skin, first-degree burns are the least severe and usually cause redness, inflammation, and soreness.

- Second-degree burns: affecting the dermis or second layer of skin, second-degree burns typically cause blistering along with the pain and redness associated with first-degree burns.
- Third-degree burns: affecting even deeper layers of the skin, third-degree burns damage the nerves, hair follicles, and even blood vessels.

✓ Good to Know

There are approximately 10,000 pediatric burn injuries annually in the United States. For children under age 2 (who account for half of all childhood burn hospitalizations), the most common burns happen to the hands and wrists from touching hot liquids or objects. After age 2, the most common burns happen in fires. Many burns are preventable.

While minor burns will usually heal within a couple of weeks, more severe burns do require medical attention and can result in scarring. Infection can also result if a burn causes a break in the skin exposing underlying layers. The treatment alternatives in this section are most effective for first- or second-degree burns.

Burns Side-by-Side Comparison

	Conventional Remedy	Treatment Alternative
Generic Treatment	Silver sulfadiazine	Aloe vera
Sample Brand Name Treatment	Silvadene	Aubrey Organic Pure Aloe

	Conventional Remedy	Treatment Alternative
How it works	Silvadene helps to kill bacteria and prevent infection in second- and third-degree burns. It also helps to treat existing infection.	Aubrey Organic Pure Aloe Vera provides natural relief to minor burns. It helps to soothe and hydrate the skin.
Dosage	Dosage must be determined by a doctor. Typical dosage for children ages 2 months and older: apply cream1-2 times daily to site of burn after cleaning the burn. Keep burn site covered in cream at all times.	For topical use only: shake bottle well and apply aloe vera to site of minor burn as needed; refrigerate after opening.
Active Ingredients	Silver sulfadiazine	*Aloe barbadensis* leaf juice, *Citrus grandis* extract, *Cyamopsis tetragonoloba* gum, tocopherol
Common Mild Side Effects	Burning, itching, pain, redness, hives, changes in skin tone	None
Less Common Serious Side Effects	Allergic reaction, difficulty urinating, fever, sore throat, jaundice, extreme fatigue, joint pain, severe rash, unexplained bruising or bleeding, nausea, vomiting, changes in mood, abdominal pain brownish-gray skin discoloration	Allergic reaction

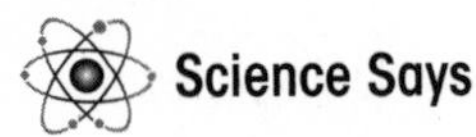

Science Says

Researchers at the Department of Surgery at the Mazandaran University of Medical Sciences in Iran studied aloe vera cream versus silver sulfadiazine cream in treating second-degree burns. In the study, 30 patients with similar second-degree burns at two different body part sites were chosen. Each patient had one burn treated with topical aloe vera cream and the other burn treated with silver sulfadiazine cream. Results showed complete healing by day 16 for burns treated with aloe vera versus 19 days for burn sites treated with the sulfadiazine cream.

Natural Selection

If aloe vera doesn't help your child, consider calendula ointment. It can help heal minor burn wounds by promoting healing and growth of the skin. Calendula ointment also prevents infection as it contains antibacterial properties. Another treatment alternative is honey. Honey can be applied topically to the burn site; its anti-inflammatory and antibacterial properties will expedite healing and reduce the risk of infection. Manuka honey from New Zealand is particularly effective for this use.

Cuts and Scrapes

A scraped knee is considered a rite of passage for kids everywhere. Falling off a bike while jumping ramps, turning the couch into an ill-advised obstacle course, sliding down banisters backwards, and other childhood daredevil moves all cause the occasional cut or scrape.

Unlike bruises, cuts and scraps involve a breaking of the skin as a result of the physical trauma associated. Skinned knees and elbows, along with paper cuts and other minor injuries, all fall into the cut and scrape category. Of course, more severe lacerations require medical attention.

Parental Guidance

"When our son was learning to walk, skinned knees were commonplace. Even walking an inch away from him couldn't prevent the unexpected tumble. Luckily, he was only two feet tall at the time and had a small distance to fall. We developed a three-step ritual for every skinned knee. First we washed the scrape under cool water, then a tender kiss landed on the injury spot, and finally, my son picked his favorite Curious George Band-Aid to cover the wound. By the time he could talk, he was reciting the three steps almost while falling down. Talk about a holistic alternative!"

—Jeff, father to 5-year-old son Gabriel

The area of a cut or scrape should be kept clean, particularly when bleeding occurs. This is the best way to avoid infection. Water and mild soap can usually help disinfect in cases of minor wounds. At times, a cut or scrape is more than just superficial and requires treatment. In these cases, one of the treatment alternatives discussed here should heal the cut or scrape quickly and get your kid back to climbing sofa cushions.

As Carrie Donegan and Elena Yorda, authors of the book *Essential Oils 101,* state, "Try to avoid using a triple antibiotic cream for minor cuts; it's like using a sledgehammer to crack a walnut. A simpler alternative, *Melaleuca alternifolia,* can be applied straight to the skin and is a natural antiseptic oil.

Cuts and Scrapes Side-by-Side Comparison

	Conventional Remedy	Treatment Alternative
Generic Treatment	Polymyxin B, bacitracin zinc, neomycin sulfate	Calendula
Sample Brand Name Treatment	Neosporin	Weleda Calendula Ointment

	Conventional Remedy	Treatment Alternative
How it works	As an antibiotic, Neosporin helps provide pain relief and helps to prevent infection at sites of injuries like minor cuts and scrapes.	This ointment helps moisturize, heal, and soothe skin problems such as irritation and damage associated with minor cuts and scrapes.
Dosage	Clean the affected area, coat the area with Neosporin, and then cover with a bandage to keep ointment in place.	Apply ointment to the affected area 3-4 times per day.
Active Ingredients	Polymyxin B, bacitracin zinc, neomycin sulfate, pramoxine	*Calendula officinalis*
Common Mild Side Effects	Minor burning, redness,	None
Less Common Serious Side Effects	Allergic reaction, severe irritation, worsened wound, redness, pain, burning, cracked skin, hearing impairment, loss of balance, changes in urination	None

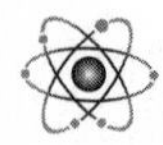

Science Says

At the Amala Cancer Research Center in Kerala, India, researchers in the Department of Biochemistry studied the wound-healing power of flower extracts from *Calendula officinalis*. For the purpose of this study, rats with excision wounds were checked. Researchers found 90 percent wound closure rates for those treated with calendula versus 51 percent in the control group after eight days. Additionally, skin regrowth occurred nearly five days faster for those rats treated with *Calendula officinalis*.

Natural Selection

As mentioned earlier in this chapter, both aloe vera and honey can help with cuts and scraps. Aloe vera naturally contains antibacterial properties to both provide relief and prevent infection. Honey naturally contains hydrogen peroxide that will help disinfect the cut or scrape site. It may also expedite the wound recovery process. If you've got onions lying around, you can chop them and mix them into the honey. Coating this mixture on your child's injury for 30 to 45 minutes can speed healing and provide pain relief.

Dehydration

Did you know the human body is comprised of more than 60 percent water? It's amazing to think dehydration is even possible. You'd think your body would have this endless supply of water waiting to rehydrate at a moment's notice. Unfortunately, it's not quite that simple. If it were, energy and electrolyte drinks wouldn't fly off the shelves.

The human body needs water to operate properly. Without enough liquids, your child can become dehydrated. Simply put, dehydration occurs when the body loses more fluids than it consumes. Water is not just about refreshment. It helps digest food properly, promotes waste elimination through urine, and even regulates body temperature. Throughout the day, fluids are routinely lost through sweating, urination, and bowel movements.

Your child's job is to replace these lost fluids throughout the day. Minerals like sodium and potassium are especially important to replace because they help to keep water inside the body's blood vessels where it belongs. Just replacing water is adequate for mild dehydration but won't do the trick for moderate or severe deficits.

The first signs of dehydration include obvious extreme thirst. Additional symptoms include lethargy, dry or sticky mouth, sunken eyes, lightheadedness, dark or decreased urine, and dizziness. When the dehydration is accompanied by vomiting, diarrhea, or decreased appetite, it's often a sign of dehydration brought on by a viral or bacterial illness. Regardless of the cause or specific symptoms, the following treatment alternatives can get that water level back over 60 percent.

Dehydration Side-by-Side Comparison

	Conventional Remedy	Treatment Alternative
Generic Treatment	Water, sucrose, dextrose, citric acid, sodium chloride (table salt), sodium citrate, monopotassium phosphate, and flavoring/coloring ingredients	Coconut water
Sample Brand Name Treatment	Gatorade Lemon-Lime Thirst Quencher	Zico Natural Bottled Pure Premium Coconut Water
How it works	Gatorade helps hydrate the body and provide it with carbs, sodium, and potassium. It replenishes electrolytes lost through exercise or other forms of dehydration. It is not recommended for babies who are still fed exclusively by formula or breast milk.	Zico Natural Bottled Pure Premium Coconut Water is made of pure coconut water and is naturally lower in calories and sodium than many sports drinks. It contains 5 electrolytes (sodium, magnesium, calcium, potassium and phosphorus) to hydrate the body.
Dosage	Drink as needed to provide fluids and electrolytes to the body. Do not exceed recommended daily values of vitamins, sodium, and sugar. Serving size is 8 ounces.	Drink as needed to hydrate the body and provide it with antioxidants and potassium. Serving size is 14 ounces.

	Conventional Remedy	Treatment Alternative
Active Ingredients	Water, sucrose syrup, glucose-fructose syrup, citric acid, salt, sodium citrate, monopotassium phosphate	100% natural coconut water from concentrate,
Common Mild Side Effects	None	None
Less Common Serious Side Effects	None (other than illness caused by overconsumption of ingredients)	Allergic reaction

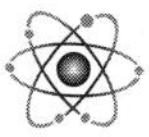

Science Says

At the Sports Science Unit at the Universiti Sains School of Medical Sciences in Malaysia, scientists studied the effectiveness of rehydration with sodium-enriched coconut water after dehydration from exercise. For the study, sodium-enriched coconut water was compared to plain water, a sports drink, and fresh young coconut water. Ten healthy male subjects were tested for whole body rehydration and plasma volume restoration after exercise-induced dehydration. After strenuous exercise, participants underwent a two-hour rehydration period drinking one of the four beverages studied. Researchers found the sodium-enriched coconut water to be equally effective to ingesting a commercial sports drink for whole-body rehydration. Furthermore, coconut water avoids unnecessary and potentially harmful artificial ingredients.

Natural Selection

If you're looking for a healthy electrolyte rehydration option, especially for infants and toddlers, consider Nature's One PediaVance, an organic alternative to Pedialyte. It can be given to your child at the first sign of dehydration and continued until a soft stool is passed (an indicator of proper rehydration). If your child won't drink the solution, you can make ice pops out of the PediaVance. Additionally, foods high in potassium (like bananas, avocados, almonds, and beans) can help restore hydration as the potassium acts as a natural electrolyte.

Hives

Medically known as urticaria, hives are a skin reaction that causes red, inflamed welts to appear on the skin.

Hives can occur anywhere on the body. Often the result of an allergic reaction, hives may also be brought on from stress or heat sensitivity. Either way, hives are an immune system response caused by histamines released whenever the body detects a foreign pathogen.

Beyond the red welts, hives also cause itchiness, stinging, and burning from the increased skin sensitivity. If you're busy right now Googling photos of the beehive hairdo, close your browser and learn about these treatment alternatives.

Hives Side-by-Side Comparison

	Conventional Remedy	Treatment Alternative
Generic Treatment	Diphenhydramine	Stinging nettle
Sample Brand Name Treatment	Benadryl Children's Allergy Liquid	Traditional Medicinals Organic Nettle Leaf Tea
How it works	Diphenhydramine is an antihistamine that helps provide relief from the symptoms associated with hives.	Traditional Medicinals Organic Nettle Leaf Tea contains nettles, which can behave as an antihistamine and help temper allergic responses such as hives.

	Conventional Remedy	Treatment Alternative
Dosage	Children ages 6 and up: take 5-10mL every 4-6 hours. Do not exceed 6 doses in 24 hours.	Not recommended for children under 12 years of age; pour 8 oz. of hot water over 1-2 tea bags. Steep for 10 minutes and sip when cooled. Drink up to 3-4 cups per day.
Active Ingredients	Diphenhydramine HCl 12.5mg	Organic nettle leaf
Common Mild Side Effects	Drowsiness, weakness, excitability, dry mouth or nose, constipation, diarrhea, headache, nausea, vomiting, decreased appetite	Mild gastrointestinal upset
Less Common Serious Side Effects	Allergic reaction, irregular heartbeat, difficulty urinating or inability to urinate, chills, fever, dizziness, seizure, severe drowsiness, tremor, changes in vision, unexplained bruising or bleeding	Allergic reaction

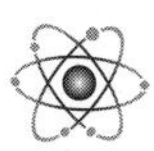

Science Says

At the HerbalScience Group in Naples, Florida, researchers studied the anti-inflammatory actions associated with nettle extract. Scientists discovered that nettle extract inhibits many of the key inflammatory mediators of seasonal allergies (including hives). Among the positives, nettle extract blocks the release of prostaglandins and histamines, pro-inflammatory chemicals that cause hay fever symptoms. This study provides a clear explanation of the mechanisms by which nettle extract can reduce allergic symptoms like hives.

Natural Selection

Hive symptoms and inflammation can be reduced with amaranth seeds. Simply prepare a tea with two tablespoons of amaranth seeds and boiling water. Have your child consume the tea after it steeps for approximately 10 minutes and after straining the seeds. Ginger can also be effective in alleviating hive symptoms, particularly itching and stinging. Mix together grated ginger and boiling water, then add the concoction to a warm bath for your child to soak for several minutes. Finally, sandalwood oil can be effective in reducing itching and speed healing if topically applied to the site of a hives outbreak.

Insect Bites

Does it ever amaze you how many insects are in existence? Have you ever been swarmed by mosquitoes and thought, "If there are fifty mosquitoes around me, and there are seven billion people on this planet, there must be 350,000,000,000 mosquitoes living on Earth!" Maybe that's not an exact count, but it doesn't even take into account flies, fleas, ticks, and horseflies.

Most common during warm weather months, an insect bite injects venom into the body causing a reaction. In most cases, the reaction is minor including skin irritation, pain, or redness. If your child is allergic to the insect bite, the reaction may turn into hives, difficulty breathing, severe swelling, abdominal pain, and nausea.

✓ Good to Know

Would you believe there are more than 10 quintillion insects in the world? That includes more than one million different insect species. It's no wonder insect bites are so common. We're simply outnumbered on this planet!

In most cases, an insect bite can be treated at home (unless you're dealing with a severe allergic reaction). The most common insect bites come from mosquitoes, flies, and ants. Spider bites are less common, and our long-legged friends aren't technically insects anyway—they're arachnids. Regardless of what bites your child, you'll want to check out these treatment options.

Insect Bites Side-by-Side Comparison

	Conventional Remedy	Treatment Alternative
Generic Treatment	Benzocaine	Baking soda
Sample Brand Name Treatment	Lanacane Anti-itch	Arm and Hammer Baking Soda
How it works	Lanacane Anti-itch is a topical anesthetic that provides temporary relief from itching caused by insect bites.	Arm and Hammer Baking Soda has alkaline properties that help neutralize a bite or sting caused by insects.
Dosage	Children under 2 years of age: consult a doctor before use; children ages 2 years and older: clean affected area and apply a small amount of Lanacane topically 1-3 times daily. Do not use for longer than 7 days.	After cleaning skin, apply topically as a paste to insect bites. To make paste, use a 3:1 ratio of baking soda to water. Apply as needed until pain and itching subside.
Active Ingredients	Benzocaine	Baking soda
Common Mild Side Effects	Mild burning, stinging, irritation, redness, or itching	Minor stinging

	Conventional Remedy	Treatment Alternative
Less Common Serious Side Effects	Allergic reaction, dizziness, irregular heartbeat, headache, fatigue, confusion, severe burning or stinging, blistering, methemoglobinemia	None

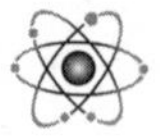

Science Says

Baking soda is a natural pH neutralizer, counteracting most acid solutions. This natural pH-neutralizing effect of baking soda makes it a perfect choice for soothing stings and bites, as many insect venoms are acidic.

Natural Selection

Aloe vera, when applied topically, can reduce the stinging sensation associated with a sting or bite. Vinegar applied directly to the bite can neutralize the pain and provide quick relief. Capsaicin (the active component in chili peppers) has been shown to block the pain and swelling caused by melittin, a major bee venom constituent. Finally, ice wrapped in a towel will reduce redness, pain, and inflammation when applied to the bite. Over the course of 1 hour, apply the ice for 15 minutes, and then break for 45 minutes. Repeat until symptoms subside.

Nosebleeds

When your toddler tumbles down the stairs or trips at the playground, you are expecting the scrape and ensuing blood. However, seeing blood pouring from a child's nose out of nowhere can surprise even the most mild-mannered parent.

Your child's nose contains many blood vessels that can rupture, which leads to bleeding. Why, exactly, do nose blood vessels rupture? A variety of factors—most of which are not considered dangerous—can cause nosebleeds. These include dry nose, nose trauma (i.e., getting hit in the nose), allergic irritation, or an infection.

In most cases, blood loss is minimal from a nosebleed and there are no accompanying symptoms. In rare cases, heavier blood loss can lead to feelings of dizziness or lightheadedness. Before the next drops of blood seep from your child's nostril, get to know these treatment alternatives.

Nosebleeds Side-by-Side Comparison

	Conventional Remedy	Treatment Alternative
Generic Treatment	Phenylephrine hydrochloride	Saline gel
Sample Brand Name Treatment	Neo-Synephrine	NeilMed NasoGel (Drip Free Gel Spray)
How it works	Neo-Synephrine is a decongestant that helps constrict blood vessels on a temporary basis. This helps to stop or reduce bleeding associated with a bloody nose.	NeilMed NasoGel helps to moisturize and lubricate the nasal passages, which can reduce or stop a nosebleed.
Dosage	Children under 12 years of age: consult a doctor prior to use; children 12 years of age and older: spray 2-3 times in each nostril every 4 hours as needed. Do not use for more than 3 days.	Use 1-2 sprays in each nostril every 4-6 hours. Consult a doctor before use in small children.

	Conventional Remedy	Treatment Alternative
Active Ingredients	Phenylephrine hydrochloride 0.5%	Sodium hyaluronate, sodium chloride, sodium bicarbonate, glycerin, aloe vera, allantoin, propylene glycol, purified water, Benzalkonium Chloride
Common Mild Side Effects	Stinging, burning, increased nasal discharge, sneezing, headache, minor dizziness	None
Less Common Serious Side Effects	Allergic reaction	Allergic reaction

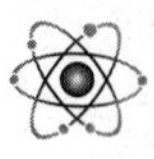

Science Says

At Mount Carmel Medical Center in Columbus, Ohio, researchers studied the effectiveness of nasal saline gel in the treatment of recurrent anterior epistaxis (bleeding from the nostrils) in anticoagulated patients (people on blood thinners at highest risk for nosebleeds). Researchers attempted to discover if the use of nasal saline gel would be an effective alternative to more invasive measures. For this open-label study, 74 patients were given the saline nasal gel to self-apply at the first sign of bleeding. At the three-month mark, the patients were checked and 93 percent had experienced a complete cessation to bleeding symptoms.

Natural Selection

Before trying any treatment, you can first pinch the base of your child's nose with the thumb and index finger for five minutes to see if the bleeding subsides. Contrary to popular belief, you should have your child put her chin to her chest and hold her head down, not up, to limit choking on bloody post-nasal drip. You can also apply ice to the bridge of your child's nose to constrict blood vessels and stop the bleeding. Persistent nosebleeds can be caused by a deficiency in vitamin C or K, which can be diagnosed by a medical professional. These vitamins can be taken in supplement form or naturally from foods. Oranges, bell peppers, and grapefruit are high in vitamin C, while leafy greens, broccoli, and kale are high in vitamin K.

Poison Ivy

Back in my grade school there was a girl named Ivy in grammar class. You'll never guess her nickname. Okay, maybe this section gives it away. That's right, everyone called her Poison Ivy. It was a real shame because she was the sweetest, most caring, friendliest girl in class. One can only blame her parents for not nickname-proofing her when selecting a first name. Or maybe they were just fans of one of Batman's archenemies.

Poison ivy is a plant that triggers an allergic reaction when touched. The allergen in poison ivy is called urushiol, and the resulting reaction from contact is called dermatitis.

✓ Good to Know

Did you know some folks are actually immune to poison ivy? That's right, these lucky ones can literally roll in it without the hint of a reaction. Before you test your own immunity, or that of your child, keep in mind you can gain or lose immunity as you age. So an itch-free roll one day may be quite the opposite situation a few years later.

If your child comes in contact with poison ivy, the telltale signs are splotchy, red, itchy bumps on the surface of the skin. Your child will likely see these bumps within two days of exposure to a poison ivy plant. Given the 48-hour lapse, you may inadvertently miscategorize this ailment if you forget where your child was two days ago. Additional symptoms include blisters that may ooze, red or flesh-colored skin bumps, and overall skin sensitivity.

In cases of a poison ivy allergy, the reaction can be more severe. Your child may experience difficulty breathing or seeing; swelling of the lips, eyelids, or throat; and more intense itchy sensations.

If your child is showing symptoms of poison ivy exposure, read about the following treatment alternatives to understand your options for soothing your child's condition.

Poison Ivy Side-by-Side Comparison

	Conventional Remedy	Treatment Alternative
Generic Treatment	Prednisolone	Kaolin, zinc oxide, tea tree oil
Sample Brand Name Treatment	Orapred	All Terrain Poison Ivy/Oak Cream
How it works	Orapred is a steroid taken orally that helps temper the body's histamine response to ailments such as poison ivy. It helps reduce inflammation, pain, and itching.	All Terrain Poison Ivy/ Oak Cream helps provide relief from poison ivy by drying out oozing and weeping associated with this ailment. It also helps prevent it from spreading if applied soon after contact with poison ivy.
Dosage	Dosage must be decided by a doctor based on severity of poison ivy and the age and weight of the child.	Apply topically as needed for treatment of poison ivy. Do not use for longer than 7 days.
Active Ingredients	Prednisolone	Kaolin clay, zinc oxide

	Conventional Remedy	Treatment Alternative
Common Mild Side Effects	Nausea, headache, dizziness, insomnia, acne, excessive sweating, bloating	None
Less Common Serious Side Effects	Allergic reaction, weight gain, changes in vision, shortness of breath, changes in mood or behavior, blood in urine or stools, muscle weakness, high blood pressure, irregular heartbeat, severe stomach or back pain, seizure, chest pain, unexplained bruising or bleeding, fever, chills, unusual hair growth	None

Natural Selection

Consider jewelweed as an herbal remedy for poison ivy; it can help relieve itching symptoms while healing the rash and can even reduce skin sensitivity. You can simply crush the leaves, mix with a small amount of water, and apply directly to the skin. Interestingly, jewelweed is typically found growing next to poison ivy. So if you accidentally touch poison ivy and you realize it, just look "next door" to find jewelweed.

And not to be forgotten, 2 to 3 drops of tea tree oil mixed with a teaspoon of a carrier oil (like grapeseed oil) will reduce redness and itching associated with poison ivy. Finally, snag some oatmeal from the kitchen cabinet and make a warm oatmeal bath for your child to soak and soothe.

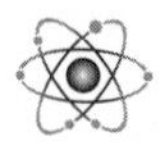

Science Says

Scientists in the Department of Dermatology at the University of California in San Francisco studied kaolin as a preventative measure for poison ivy. Kaolin was found to be 95 percent effective in protecting against poison ivy outbreaks. For poison ivy that was already contracted, tea tree oil was studied for treating the itching sensation by researchers at Skane University Hospital in Sweden. Researchers in the Department of Dermatology found the tea tree oil to be an effective anti-itch agent for those experiencing symptoms associated with poison ivy.

Sprains

We sure do need our wrists, ankles, and knees to get through the day. These body parts are critical for walking, changing direction, picking stuff up, and climbing. It's no wonder sprains are so common. How can any body part be expected to perform so many actions and not twist or tear here and there?

A sprain is an injury to a muscle or tendon that typically includes a stretch or tear of the ligament (a band of tissue that connects bones or links joints). Sprains can occur anytime, caused by anything from exercise to an unexpected fall.

If your child sprains a body part, he'll feel localized pain at the site of the sprain and possibly swelling, bruising, or decreased mobility. In many cases, you'll wonder if it's a sprain or a break and need to seek medical attention (including an x-ray) for official confirmation.

Once you know it's a sprain, not a fracture or break, consider these treatments to get your child back on her feet again (unless, of course, it's a sprained wrist).

Sprains Side-by-Side Comparison

	Conventional Remedy	Treatment Alternative
Generic Treatment	Naproxen	Comfrey extract
Sample Brand Name Treatment	Aleve	Burt's Bees Res-Q Ointment
How it works	Aleve contains naproxen, which provides temporary relief from pain caused by injuries like a sprain.	Burt's Bees Res-Q Ointment uses herbal ingredients to topically treat symptoms of an injury such as a sprain. Ointment helps expedite healing and promote new cell growth.
Dosage	Children under 12 years of age: consult a doctor prior to use; children 12 and older: take 1 tablet every 8-12 hours as needed. Do not exceed 2 tablets in 8-12 hours or 3 tablets in 24 hours. Drink 8 oz. of water with tablet.	Apply a thin layer of ointment topically after site of injury is cleaned 2 times per day until symptoms subside.
Active Ingredients	Naproxen	Comfrey
Common Mild Side Effects	Diarrhea, dizziness, upset stomach, mild heartburn, constipation, gas, bloating	None
Less Common Serious Side Effects	Allergic reaction, vomiting blood, black or bloody stools, faintness, severe stomach or abdominal pain, stiff neck, changes in behavior, jaundice, changes in hearing, swelling, weight gain, changes in urination, changes in vision	Allergic reaction

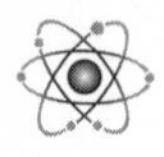

Science Says

Comfrey is known in folk medicine as knitbone based on its traditional use in healing fractures. The herb's mechanism of action is now thought to be via allantoin, a constituent that speeds up the natural replacement of bone cells. At the Istituto Ortopedico Galeazzi in Italy, researchers compared comfrey extract to a nonsteroidal anti-inflammatory drug (NSAID) in the treatment of sprains; 82 patients received comfrey extract while 82 received an NSAID. Comfrey extract was superior to the NSAID in relieving pain, swelling, and tenderness. It is very important to note that comfrey is safe for external use only and should not be taken internally as it can cause severe liver toxicity.

Natural Selection

Bromelain, an enzyme naturally found in pineapple, can help reduce the swelling and inflammation associated with sprains. And no matter what else you do, standard sprain guidance involves RICE. We're not talking about eating spoonfuls of the grain; rather, we're referring to the RICE acronym:

- R = Rest: avoid putting pressure on the sprained body part, as rest will ensure proper healing.
- I = Ice: apply ice for 15 minutes every 1 to 2 hours to relieve swelling and bruising symptoms.
- C = Compression: wrap or bandage the sprained body part to reduce swelling and promote proper and faster healing.
- E = Elevation: elevate the sprained body part to promote proper draining of fluid buildup.

Sunburn

"Don't forget to put on sunscreen!" What parent hasn't shouted these words as their child flies out the door for a day at the beach with friends? If only children could be instantly sprayed with full-body sunscreen the moment they cross the threshold of your doorway to the outside, melanoma could be forced into near extinction.

Sunburn refers to skin damage caused by exposure to the sun's ultraviolet rays. Sunscreen, hats, and proper sunny-weather attire are the best protectors against sunburn. Your child's likelihood of sunburn goes beyond sunscreen and attire, however. Fair-skinned kids and those with red or blonde hair are more susceptible to damage from ultraviolet rays.

✓ Good to Know

Sunscreen is classified by strength or SPF, which stands for Sun Protection Factor. SPF numbers typically range from as low as 2 all the way past 60. These numbers refer to the product's ability to block out the sun's burning rays. At an SPF of 2, only 50 percent of the sun's harmful rays are blocked out. At SPF ratings of 15 or higher, more than 93 percent of the sun's rays are stopped.

Common symptoms of sunburn include red skin that feels hot and is sensitive to the touch. Beyond the uncomfortable feeling of the skin itself, your child may also experience minor dizziness, low-grade fever, blistering, and nausea.

If your child just returned from the beach looking redder than a Maine lobster, run out to the store for one of these treatment options. His skin will thank you later!

Sunburn Side-by-Side Comparison

	Conventional Remedy	Treatment Alternative
Generic Treatment	Benzocaine	Aloe vera, vitamin E, vitamin C
Sample Brand Name Treatment	Solarcaine Spray	Jason Aloe Vera 84% Moisturizing Cream
How it works	Solarcaine contains lidocaine and aloe vera to help soothe skin and cool the skin. It also adds moisture to the skin.	Jason Aloe Vera 84% Moisturizing Cream helps soothe, hydrate, and repair skin that is damaged by sunburn.
Dosage	Children under 2: consult a doctor prior to use; children ages 2 and up: apply spray topically 3-4 times per day as needed for relief. Use should not exceed 7 days.	Apply topically several times per day or as needed while sunburn symptoms persist.
Active Ingredients	Benzocaine	Aloe vera, herbal extracts, vitamin A, vitamin C, and vitamin E
Common Mild Side Effects	Minor pain or tingling	None
Less Common Serious Side Effects	Allergic reaction, severe skin irritation, extreme fatigue, methemoglobinemia	Allergic reaction

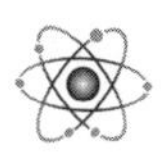

Science Says

Vitamins C and E combine as an effective treatment for sunburn according to scientists at Dermatologische Klinik und Poliklinik der Ludwig-Maximilians-Universität München in Munich, Germany. In their study, participants took either a placebo or 2 grams of vitamin C combined with 1,000 IU of vitamin E. Sunburn reactions were checked before and after eight days of treatment. Researchers found vitamin C and E effectively reduced the sunburn reaction which may also indicate a subsequent reduced risk of UV-induced skin damage. In a separate study at the Pharmacy Practice Unit at Naresuan University in Phitsanulok, Thailand, researchers examined the efficacy of aloe vera for burn wound healing. As discussed previously in this chapter, aloe vera was shown to promote faster healing while soothing burn symptoms.

Natural Selection

Calendula ointment can be applied topically to promote new skin growth and expedite healing after sunburn. A bath with chamomile tea also provides natural sunburn relief. Simply steep 4-5 bags of chamomile tea in boiling water and add to the bath for a soak and soothe session. Finally, five drops of lavender oil added to a teaspoon of water or aloe can be gently applied to sunburn areas to reduce inflammation and improve pain symptoms.

Spotlight On: Aloe

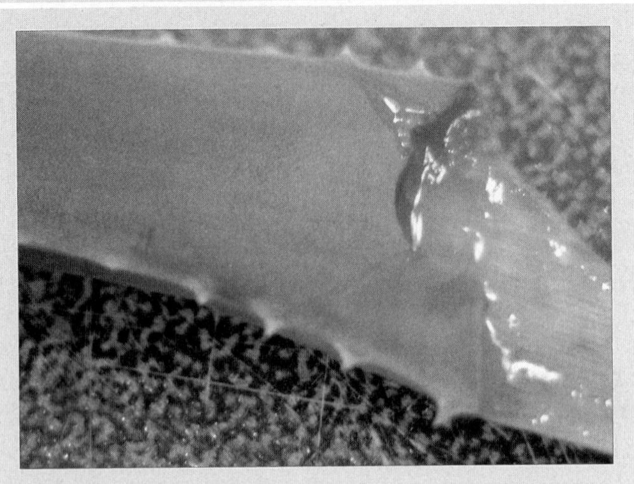

The gelatinous interior of an aloe vera leaf.

Aloe vera popped up all over this chapter on first aid for bumps, burns, bruises, and bites. In fact, it was so popular throughout this chapter as a treatment alternative, it deserves its own spotlight.

Would you believe aloe vera usage can be traced back over 6,000 years ago to early Egypt, where the plant was seen on stone carvings? At that time, aloe vera was known as the plant of immortality and was typically presented as a burial gift for deceased pharaohs.

We've seen in this chapter that aloe vera is commonly used topically to treat a variety of wounds, burns, and skin conditions. That explains why it's such a popular ingredient in hundreds of skin products. According to the Natural Comprehensive Medicines Database, aloe gel contains numerous active factors that block pain, itching, and inflammation while increasing microcirculation to speed healing of wounds and burns. Finally, aloe gel seems to possess potent antibacterial and antifungal properties.

11

Aches and Pains

"You can make your own aromatherapy rub to soothe those aching muscles. Take one tablespoon of almond or olive oil and add the following essential oils: four drops chamomile, four drops rosemary, and four drops lavender. Mix well and rub into sore muscles. Avoid getting in eyes. And remember, arnica is the go-to herb for strains, sprains, and bruises. There are numerous arnica salves and ointments in the marketplace. Apply as directed. Just remember, don't use on open cuts or wounds."

—Tieraona Low Dog, MD—Fellowship Director, Arizona Center for Integrative Medicine; Clinical Associate Professor of Medicine, University of Arizona Health Sciences, Arizona Center for Integrative Medicine

Pain, pain, go away; please come back another day. Might this be the mantra of any child experiencing aches and pains? If you're a child of the 1980s, you probably remember the show *Growing Pains* with Kirk Cameron. Airing for seven years from 1985 to 1992, the show featured a working mother and stay-at-home psychiatrist father together raising three kids. Thanks to a sitcom writing team, the growing pains were guaranteed in every episode.

Your child doesn't need a television deal to experience aches and pains, including growing pains, joint pains, and muscle aches. With so many bones, muscles, and joints in the human body, it's no wonder something can break down. Come to think of it, the human body is quite amazing for not acting up more often. If your child is experiencing any of the aches and pains just described, read on for conventional and natural remedies galore. The sooner you learn about these treatment alternatives, the sooner your child can replace "pain" with "rain" in the song.

Growing Pains

Growing up is hard enough without experiencing pain along the way. Children need to learn to read, walk, talk, play with others, feed themselves, drive a car, and get a job. We could spend this entire chapter listing skills your child will need to navigate this world. Let's get through growing pains before worrying about your child's first job!

While the specific cause of growing pains is still a mystery, it is believed to be associated with rapid growth of bones, tendons and ligaments during growth spurts. This quick gain in height may contribute to growing pains. It's also possible these pains stem from high levels of activity resulting in muscle soreness.

The President of the Pediatrics Council of the American Chiropractic Association, Elise G. Hewitt, DC, had the following to say on growing pains:

> "Growing pains is actually a misnomer—it doesn't hurt to grow. Growing pains are usually the result of referred pain secondary to locking of skeletal joints in the lower spine and pelvis. This locking irritates local nerves, which the body interprets as coming from a site further down the path of the nerve, causing children to feel pain in their legs and/or feet. Chiropractors use manual therapies to restore normal function in the affected spinal and pelvic joints, thus stopping the nerve irritation and relieving the growing pains."

So while the cause might still be mysterious, the most common site for growing pains is in one or both legs, typically from the knees through the calves. Although growing pains can strike anytime, nighttime hours are usually prime time for the pain. Minor headache or stomachache can also accompany growing pains. If your child is asking why it hurts to grow, then these remedies are worth a look.

Growing Pains Side-by-Side Comparison

	Conventional Remedy	Treatment Alternative
Generic Treatment	Acetaminophen	Vitamin D
Sample Brand Name Treatment	Children's Tylenol Liquid Suspension	Carlson Super Daily D_3 Drops
How it works	Children's Tylenol temporarily relieves pain such as that associated with childhood growth and growing pains.	Vitamin D is essential for healthy growth. Growing pains may be reduced or eliminated if a child gets an adequate amount of vitamin D.
Dosage	Under 24 lbs/under 2 years: consult doctor; 24-35 lbs/2-3 years: 1 tsp or 5mL; 36-47 lbs/4-5 years: 1.5 tsp or 7.5mL; 48-59 lbs/6-8 years: 2 tsp or 10mL; 60-71 lbs/9-10 years: 2.5 tsp or 12.5mL; 72-95 lbs/11 years: 3 tsp or 15mL; repeat dose every 4 hours as needed; do not exceed 5 doses in 24 hours.	Children ages 2 and up: take one drop daily. May be mixed into food or drink or taken from a spoon (1,000 IU daily).
Active Ingredients	Acetaminophen	Vitamin D_3
Common Mild Side Effects	Constipation, diarrhea, drowsiness, trouble sleeping	None
Less Common Serious Side Effects	Allergic reaction, liver damage, stomach pain, dizziness, changes in vision, irregular heartbeat, difficulty urinating	Associated with vitamin D overdose: nausea, headache, vomiting, stomach pain, dizziness, fatigue, weakness, decreased appetite, insomnia

Science Says

Researchers at the Department of Pediatrics at Liaquat National Medical College and Hospital in Karachi studied vitamin D levels in children with growing pains. Their goal was to determine the relationship between those children experiencing growing pains and their associated vitamin D levels. For the study, 100 children ages 5 to 12 who cited limb pain (thereby fulfilling the diagnostic definition of growing pains) were included. Overall, only 6 percent of participants in the study showed normal levels of vitamin D in their systems, many fewer than the general age-matched population.

Natural Selection

Gently massaging the calves or other areas of leg pain can ease discomfort from growing pains. You can use a few drops of lavender essential oil mixed with a tablespoon of massage oil to help relax your child. Warmth, either from a heating pad or hot water bottle, can help soothe leg aches. Finally, consider guided imagery to help your child overcome growing pains. The goal is to promote feelings of relaxation and relieve pain and tension. Focusing on breathing and stretching the body can increase relaxation and soothe achy muscles. Again, aromatherapy with soothing oils may be a nice complement.

Joint Pains

Ever wonder what helps your bones move in so many directions? The title of this section is a big clue! That's right, our joints are what allow us to jump and dance and generally move our skeletons in all sorts of fun ways. When it comes to joint pain, it's usually triggered by an injury, inflammation, or infection.

The most common injuries that cause joint pain include broken bones, torn ligaments, torn tendons, and sprains. Certain rare childhood illnesses can lead to joint pain, too, including sickle cell anemia, juvenile arthritis, lupus, and fibromyalgia.

✓ Good to Know

The human body has three main types of joints. Ball-and-socket joints have the greatest range of motion (for example, where the upper arm bone fits into the shoulder blade socket). Hinge joints, as found in the elbow, fingers, and toes, allow movement in only one direction. Finally, gliding joints (such as the wrist and ankle joints) are built for sideways movement. It is estimated that humans have about 250 joints in their bodies.

In many cases, particularly for injuries, joint pain is temporary and alleviates as the body self-heals. Too much movement and exertion will likely exacerbate the condition. The following remedies may also help soothe joint pain.

Joint Pains Side-by-Side Comparison

	Conventional Remedy	Treatment Alternative
Generic Treatment	Ibuprofen	Boswellia
Sample Brand Name Treatment	Children's Advil Suspension Liquid	Pure Encapsulations Boswellia AKBA
How it works	Children's Advil is a temporary pain reliever that works with the brain and nervous system to decrease the body's perception of pain.	Boswellia AKBA is an herbal supplement that helps to preserve joint cartilage and promotes healthy joints.

	Conventional Remedy	Treatment Alternative
Dosage	Under 24 lbs/under 2 years: consult doctor; 24-35 lbs/2-3 years: 1 tsp or 5mL; 36-47 lbs/4-5 years: 1.5 tsp or 7.5mL; 48-59 lbs/6-8 years: 2 tsp or 10mL; 60-71 lbs/9-10 years: 2.5 tsp or 12.5mL; 72-95 lbs/11 years: 3 tsp or 15mL; repeat dose every 6-8 hours as needed; do not exceed 4 doses in 24 hours.	Use in children: take only as directed by a doctor. Typical dosage is one capsule per day with food.
Active Ingredients	Ibuprofen	*Boswellia serrata* extract, vitamin C
Common Mild Side Effects	Constipation, diarrhea nausea, upset stomach, heartburn, headache, dizziness, drowsiness, insomnia, gas,	None
Less Common Serious Side Effects	Allergic reaction, severe vomiting or diarrhea, stiff neck, irregular heartbeat, changes in behavior, changes in urine, black or bloody stools, changes in vision or hearing, unexplained bruising or bleeding, yellowing skin or eyes, liver disease, loss of appetite, numbness, seizure, swelling or sudden weight gain	Diarrhea, rash, nausea, heartburn

Science Says

Researchers at the Cellular and Molecular Biology Division at the Laila Impex R&D Center in India completed a controlled study of the effectiveness and safety of 5-Loxin, an extract from the Boswellia tree, in the treatment of osteoarthritis of the knee. It was determined that 5-Loxin both reduces pain and improves physical functioning for patients experiencing osteo-arthritis and is safe for human consumption. The boswellia extract found in 5-Loxin is the same extract found in Pure Encapsulations recommended in this section. Boswellia has been demonstrated to be safe and effective for children for a variety of inflammatory conditions.

Natural Selection

Consider applying Topricin, a topical cream, to the site of joint pain. Topricin contains homeopathic medicines that can heal joint injuries while soothing associated joint pain. Another option is turmeric; it contains the chemical curcumin, a natural anti-inflammatory agent. It's thought to help relieve joint pain when taken orally as a supplement. Finally, a daily dose of apple cider vinegar (two tablespoons) mixed with 12 ounces of water can gradually soothe joint pain inflammation.

Muscle Aches

Muscles are associated with strength and vitality. Why else would 5-year-olds flex their biceps after a heated game of tee ball? Come to think of it, many adults do the same macho muscle flexing when successfully throwing a crumpled paper into the wastebasket from 12 feet away.

These symbols of strength can also break down—that's where muscle aches enter the picture. Described as soreness or discomfort in the body's muscles, aches can stem from injury, disease, infection, overexertion, and even muscular or neurological conditions. The pain can be localized (from a muscle strain or injury) or across the body (in cases of illness).

✓ Good to Know

With more than 650 muscles in the human body, it's no wonder folks spend so much time at the gym. There are three types of muscles: skeletal, smooth, and cardiac. Skeletal muscle is considered voluntary; you control these muscles for everyday tasks like walking. Smooth muscle is considered involuntary and includes those found within walls of organs and structures such as the stomach and bladder. Cardiac muscle refers to the heart.

Muscle aches often come along with additional ailments like bruising and swelling from an injury. This is most common in cases of sports injuries or ligament and tendon sprains from a fall or accident. Many illnesses can induce muscle aches, including Lyme disease, influenza, and fibromyalgia. In these cases, additional symptoms such as fever, weakness, fatigue, and chills can accompany the muscle aches.

For most simple muscle aches, various treatment alternatives can soothe the aches and get your child back in the game in no time. Check out the most common conventional and natural alternatives here.

Muscle Aches Side-by-Side Comparison

	Conventional Remedy	Treatment Alternative
Generic Treatment	Naproxen	*Arnica montana*
Sample Brand Name Treatment	Aleve	Boiron Arnica Gel
How it works	Aleve contains naproxen, which provides temporary relief from pain caused by muscle aches or injuries like a sprain.	Boiron Arnica Gel helps temporarily relieve pain associated with muscle aches and stiffness through the use of homeopathic ingredients. It also reduces swelling.

	Conventional Remedy	Treatment Alternative
Dosage	Children under 12 years of age: consult a doctor prior to use; children and older: take 1 tablet every 8-12 hours as needed. Do not exceed 2 tablets in 8-12 hours or 3 tablets in 24 hours. Drink 8 oz. of water with tablet	Apply a thin layer of gel topically at the first sign of muscle aches. Repeat as needed up to 3 times per day.
Active Ingredients	Naproxen	*Arnica montana* 1X HPUS
Common Mild Side Effects	Diarrhea, dizziness, upset stomach, mild heartburn, constipation, gas, bloating	Skin irritation
Less Common Serious Side Effects	Allergic reaction, vomiting blood, black or bloody stools, faintness, severe stomach or abdominal pain, stiff neck, changes in behavior, jaundice, changes in hearing, swelling, weight gain, changes in urination, changes in vision	Allergic reaction

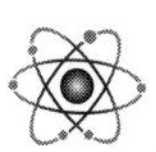

Science Says

Researchers at Freiburg University in Germany studied *Arnica montana* to uncover the root of its anti-inflammatory effects. In performing their research, scientists found a significant amount of helenalin, a naturally occurring compound that has major immune suppressant and anti-inflammatory properties.

Natural Selection

Vitamin C supplements have been known to help reduce muscle pain. When taken before or after workouts, muscle pain can be minimized, particularly for injuries associated with exercising. An herbal compress also will relieve muscle pain. Simply soak a washcloth in chamomile or ginger tea, then apply the compress to the pain site. Keep the compress in place for approximately 60 minutes.

Spotlight On: Arnica

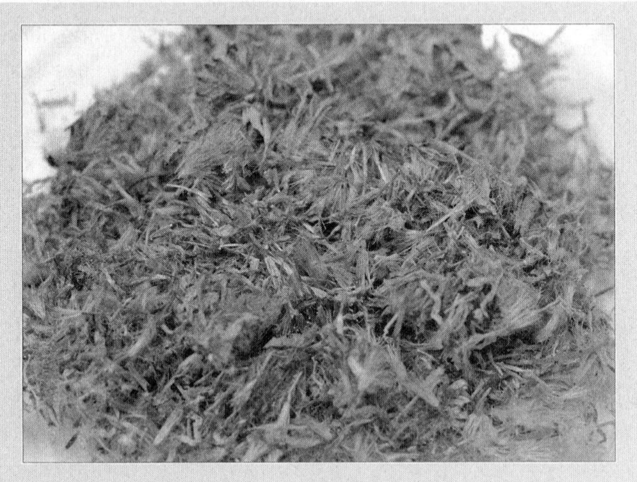

Unprocessed arnica montana.

"Homeopathic medicines work with the body's own innate healing systems to restore balance, thus avoiding unintended side effects that often come along with using pharmaceuticals. I have seen dramatic benefits in my patients from this very simple and gentle approach, and I find that with a little education, parents can be empowered to take an active role in supporting their children through times of illness."

—Heather A. Jeney, MD, The Whole Child Center

Arnica montana is a plant native to mountainous areas of both Europe and North America. It is believed that these plants contain numerous compounds with anti-inflammatory properties. That explains why it's a popular choice—both topically in mildly diluted forms and homeopathically—to relieve muscle soreness, strains, and joint pain.

Arnica typically falls under the category of homeopathic remedies. Homeopathy refers to stimulating the body's ability to heal itself through small doses of highly diluted natural substances. The principle at work is that "like cures like" so disease can be cured through substances that produce similar symptoms in non-diluted doses in healthy people. First described by Samuel Hahnemann in the early 1800s, homeopathy is an entire branch of medicine with unique practices and principles.

This principle of dilution states that the lower the medication dose, the better its effectiveness. That's why homeopathic remedies are diluted in steps and shaken thoroughly after each dilution. The process is believed to transmit energy from the original substance to the diluted remedy. This diluted remedy then stimulates the body to heal itself. This may sound unscientific, at least in terms of how we typically explain Western medicine. Interestingly, there have been numerous studies showing the homeopathic medicines have a power above and beyond a placebo effect.

Many homeopathic remedies, including arnica, come in tablet form. These pellets are typically dissolved under the tongue for maximal effect. Arnica can also be applied topically in a relatively mildly diluted form for similar effect.

12

Nervous System Worries

"Most kids with vocal or motor tics find that tics tend to be more prominent at times of emotional arousal—excitement, surprise, anger, stress, worries, etc. Helping them to understand the signals of stress and then giving them skills to modulate their own automatic nervous system activity to rebalance is very helpful. With regular practice of techniques such as meditation and biofeedback, kids can reset their ANS (Autonomic Nervous System) activity to a lower, more balanced baseline, thus promoting less overall tic activity day to day."

—Timothy Culbert, MD, FAAP, Medical Director of Pediatric Integrative Medicine, Ridgeview/Two Twelve Medical Center

The human head sure comes up in conversation a lot. There are so many well-known phrases: get a head start, we're making headway, head of the class, and (a personal favorite) head over heels. The head also houses the brain, so its all-important status is not likely to change anytime soon.

Sometimes the head becomes more of a headache, so to speak. Various ailments associated with the head and nervous system can range from temporary inconveniences like tension headaches to life-threatening conditions like seizures and epilepsy.

Luckily the treatment alternatives discussed in this chapter have shown remarkable results in improving the symptoms of these ailments, as well as decreasing the frequency and pain associated with each.

Migraine Headache

Everyone gets headaches from time to time, but migraines are not your typical ones. These severe headaches can cause other symptoms including flashes or dark spots, blurred vision, light sensitivity, numbness, nausea, and vomiting. Lasting from several hours to several days, migraine headaches can truly be debilitating.

During migraines, blood vessels in the brain spasm and chemicals are thought to be emitted from overexcited nerves surrounding the cells.

✓ Good to Know

According to the National Headache Foundation, kids are more likely to suffer migraine headaches if they have a relevant family history. In fact, nearly 30 million Americans of all ages suffer from migraines. Females are three times more likely than males to experience migraines. Some children suffer from a version called abdominal migraine in which abdominal pain and vomiting are more prominent than headache.

Research is inconclusive on the cause of migraine headaches, but there are known triggers that lead to migraines in those prone to this ailment. Common triggers include environmental changes (such as warm weather), strong scents from perfumes and colognes, menstrual cycles (for females), stress, sleeping or eating pattern changes, and even reactions to certain foods and beverages (especially meats and cheeses).

If your child has more than the typical garden-variety headache, it may be a migraine. As severe as they can be, migraines are more effectively prevented than treated in most cases. In these cases, check out the following conventional and alternative prevention remedies to prevent migraines.

Migraine Headache Side-by-Side Comparison

	Conventional Remedy	Treatment Alternative
Generic Treatment	Topiramate	Butterbur
Sample Brand Name Treatment	Topamax	Petadolex
How it works	Topamax is a daily medication taken by prescription aimed to reduce the occurrence of migraines. This is thought to be done by calming nerve cells that are prone to becoming overexcited during a migraine.	Petadolex gelcaps are an herbal supplement containing butterbur, which is a natural ingredient that can help prevent migraines. It helps with muscle tone and blood flow in the brain's blood vessels.
Dosage	A medical professional determines the dosage for each patient based upon age and need. The dosage typically begins low and increases as necessary.	Children under 6: do not use; children 6-9: consult a physician; children ages 10-17: take 1 50mg gelcap 2 times per day or as directed by a doctor.
Active Ingredients	Topiramate	Butterbur
Common Mild Side Effects	Fatigue, numbness or tingling, weight loss, change in taste, difficulty with memory or concentration, diarrhea, nausea, upper respiratory tract infection, nervousness	None

	Conventional Remedy	Treatment Alternative
Less Common Serious Side Effects	Allergic reaction, serious or permanent changes in vision, fever, decreased sweating, bones that become soft or brittle, fatigue, decreased appetite, irregular heartbeat, stunted growth, change in behavior or thought process, anxiety, depression, vomiting, suicidal thoughts, severe nausea	Allergic reaction

Science Says

Researchers in Hamburg, Germany, conducted a study with butterbur root extract to test its effectiveness in migraine prevention. In the study, 108 children and adolescents between the ages of 6 and 17 were included. Participants all reported suffering migraine headaches for at least one year. Each patient was treated with 50 to 150 milligrams (depending on age) of butterbur root extract for a period of four months. 91 percent of patients felt substantially or slightly better after four months of treatment. Researchers concluded that butterbur root extract shows potential in treating migraines and is well tolerated by children and teenagers.

Natural Selection

Magnesium, as noted by Tieraona Low Dog, MD, may help prevent migraine headaches in children.

> "Young or old, magnesium is one of the first preventive treatments for migraine I reach for. There are powdered magnesium products in the marketplace that can be blended with food or made into a fizzy drink. The dose is 200 to 400 milligrams per day based upon age."

A medical professional should choose the appropriate dosage. Instead of supplements, magnesium can also be consumed naturally in foods like nuts, brown rice, and squash. Another supplement that can help decrease migraine frequency is CoQ10. This supplemental enzyme can help promote optimal mitochodrial function. Acupuncture has been shown to reduce the frequency of migraines and may reduce the need for migraine medication. Finally, elimination diets removing potential offending foods like dairy or chocolate may be helpful.

Seizures

Watching your child have a seizure can be frightening. Your child literally loses temporary control of his body and experiences convulsions. This is a neurological problem that stems from unusual electric activity in the brain. Lasting from several seconds to several minutes, seizures can be accompanied by a loss of muscle control and even loss of consciousness.

For children, seizures may or may not be life threatening. Grand mal seizures, those with extreme convulsions and loss of consciousness, can be very serious. Less severe seizures can be triggered by something as simple as a high fever in a vulnerable child. These febrile seizures are not associated with long-term consequences and usually spontaneously resolve by age six at the latest.

Repeated seizures are typically known as epilepsy. Abnormal electrical signals sent out by the brain cause the repeated and unpredictable seizures. Triggers vary and can include fever, flashing lights, or pharmaceutical agents.

If your child is prone to seizures, read on to learn about conventional remedies and treatment alternatives that can ameliorate the symptoms and reduce seizure frequency. Given how serious seizures can be, it is very important to note that you should work closely with a specialist to determine the best course of action. Medication may be lifesaving in some cases and one should never discontinue antiseizure medications without consulting a physician.

Seizures Side-by-Side Comparison

	Conventional Remedy	Treatment Alternative
Generic Treatment	Oxcarbazepine	EEG biofeedback
Sample Brand Name Treatment	Trileptal	Neurofeedback
How it works	Trileptal is a prescription medication used to control seizures by limiting abnormal activity in the brain that may lead to seizures.	Sensors or electrodes are placed on the scalp to monitor activity of the brain. Activity that needs to be changed is addressed and healthy brain activity is also noted.
Dosage	Dosage is determined by the patient's weight and age. Common dosage is 8 mg/kg given twice daily.	The decision to use neurofeedback is determined by a doctor and must also be administered by a specially trained doctor.
Active Ingredients	Oxcarbazepine	N/A

	Conventional Remedy	Treatment Alternative
Common Mild Side Effects	Drowsiness, dizziness, diarrhea, constipation, nausea, stomach pain, vomiting, headache, changes in vision, heartburn, urinary tract infection, changes in behavior, decreased appetite, tremor, coughing	None
Less Common Serious Side Effects	Allergic reaction, worsened seizures, major vision changes, changes in urination, fever, chills, muscle pain, insomnia, decreased coordination, changes in mood, yellowing of the skin or eyes, unusual bruising or bleeding, weakness, extreme fatigue, hallucinations, suicidal ideation, muscle spasms or cramps	Skin sensitivity at the site of sensors, dizziness, fatigue, drowsiness, minor tingling, changes in behavior

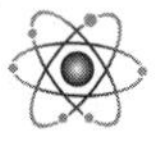

Science Says

Researchers at the Baylor College of Medicine in Houston, Texas, studied the effectiveness of electroencephalographic (EEG) biofeedback (or neurofeedback) in treating epilepsy. In this publication, researchers noted that nearly 33 percent of patients with epilepsy fail to benefit from medical treatment. In these cases, scientists meta-analyzed existing research on neurofeedback for seizure disorder for studies between 1970 and 2005. Across the studies, 74 percent of patients reported fewer weekly seizures in response to EEG biofeedback. EEG biofeedback is sometimes used as a complement or alternative to medication.

Natural Selection

Similar to its use for migraine headaches, acupuncture may be effective in decreasing the occurrence and severity of seizures. Further, acupuncture can decrease reliance on antiseizure medications. Also consider a ketogenic diet if your child suffers from seizures. This diet is extremely low in carbohydrates, moderate in protein, and very high in fat; it can help some seizure sufferers. Consult with an experienced nutritionist if you are considering the ketogenic diet. Finally, increasing omega-3 intake may benefit the nervous system and reduce seizure frequency. Omega-3s can be taken in supplement form or naturally in foods like salmon and walnuts. Remember, for children with seizures, all of these treatments should be considered only under the close supervision of your doctor.

Tension Headache

The most common form of headache is the tension headache. Pain anywhere on the forehead, side, or back of head is the telltale sign. Usually fatigue and tenderness near the eyes, neck, and scalp accompany a tension headache.

✓ Good to Know

How can you tell the difference between a migraine and tension headache? First, migraine pain is typically localized near the eye on one affected side while tension headache pain is more generalized. Further, deep throbbing and pulsating pain is common with migraines while tension headache pain is duller and more pressure-like. Finally, symptoms such as vomiting and light sensitivity are associated more with migraines than tension headaches.

Most researchers believe tension headaches are triggered by stress or changes to sleep patterns, eating or drinking habits, or even pressure or altitude-related changes. While most tension headaches improve within six hours, they can last longer. Episodes can be an independent ailment from a temporary stressor or associated with a deeper neurological condition worth investigating.

If your child is experiencing tension headaches, check out the treatment options in this section. It's a surefire ticket to easing the pain and keeping homework and a clean room on track!

Tension Headache Side-by-Side Comparison

	Conventional Remedy	Treatment Alternative
Generic Treatment	Ibuprofen	Acupuncture
Sample Brand Name Treatment	Children's Motrin	N/A
How it works	Children's Motrin temporarily relieves aches and pains such as those associated with a tension headache for up to 8 hours.	Acupuncture is a natural treatment for tension headaches that involves the use of thin needles at strategic points of the body in an effort to restore balance in the body and reduce the occurrence of tension headaches.
Dosage	Under 2 years old: ask a doctor; 24-35 lbs/2-3 years: 1 tsp; 36-47 lbs/4-5 years: 1.5 tsp; 48-59 lbs/6-8 years: 2 tsp; 60-71 lbs/9-10 years: 2.5 tsp; 72-95 lbs/11 years: 3 tsp. Repeat as needed every 6-8 hours. Do not exceed 4 doses per day.	Acupuncture should be performed only by a professional. Treatment is determined based upon individual need.
Active Ingredients	Ibuprofen	N/A

	Conventional Remedy	Treatment Alternative
Common Mild Side Effects	Drowsiness, dizziness, nausea, vomiting, diarrhea, constipation, headache, upset stomach	Tingling skin sensation, minor bleeding at the needle sites
Less Common Serious Side Effects	Allergic reaction, unexplained bruises or bleeding, changes in mood, hearing or vision impairment, stiffness, unusual weight gain, jaundice, dark urine, chest pain, fainting, irregular heartbeat, extreme fatigue or dizziness, dark vomit	None

Science Says

Researchers at the Center for Complementary Medicine Research in Munich, Germany, studied the effectiveness of acupuncture in treating tension-type headaches. All together, scientists reviewed 11 trials covering 2,317 participants. In summarizing the trials, researchers found both clinically relevant and statistically significant short-term (for three months) benefits for acupuncture versus a control group. Both pain intensity and number of headache days decreased for those receiving acupuncture. In conclusion, researchers believe acupuncture to be a viable non-pharmacological tool for patients suffering chronic or frequent episodic tension-type headaches.

Natural Selection

For tension headaches, consider mind-body therapies like biofeedback or hypnosis, targeting muscle relaxation in the face, scalp, and neck. These three areas can reduce the sensation of a tension headache. Yoga can also reduce tension headaches by engaging the mind and body.

Finally, massage is known to reduce the severity of tension headaches by relieving tense and overworked muscles.

Tics/Tourette's Syndrome

Tourette's syndrome is a neurological condition that causes uncontrollable physical displays of tics. These are quick and repetitive motor movements or vocalizations beyond the control of your child.

Researchers have been unable to pinpoint the specific cause of Tourette's syndrome, though it does appear to be passed on in families. Much more common than Tourette's syndrome are simple motor tics that occur for short periods of time, especially under stressful conditions. Also, streptococcal infections are known triggers of tics associated with obsessive-compulsive behaviors under the heading of PANDAS, or Pediatric Autoimmune Neuropsychiatric Disorders Associated with Streptococcal Infections. It is unknown how many children with tics are suffering from PANDAS, and it is believed that other infections can also cause acute onset of tics.

Tourette's syndrome usually first appears in childhood. While months may pass with no symptoms, tics can appear suddenly out of nowhere. This ailment may also be chronic; in these cases, it can regularly affect speech and motor movements.

Sudden jerking of the head, body, or arms is a common symptom of Tourette's syndrome. Additional symptoms include repetitive vocal noises (particularly including inappropriate words), strained facial expressions, compulsive movements (e.g., blinking), and even self-harm (e.g., slapping oneself). If your child has been diagnosed with Tourette's syndrome, you'll want to learn about the treatment options covered in this section.

Tics/Tourette's Syndrome Side-by-Side Comparison

	Conventional Remedy	Treatment Alternative
Generic Treatment	Guanfacine	Hypnosis
Sample Brand Name Treatment	Tenex	N/A
How it works	Tenex is a medicine designed to lower high blood pressure. In addition, it can reduce the frequency of tics associated with Tourette's syndrome.	Hypnosis can help to reduce tics associated with Tourette's syndrome by encouraging the body to use self-control and concentration, in addition to relaxation, to help manage undesired behaviors such as tics.
Dosage	Tenex should be taken daily as prescribed by a doctor to alleviate tics. Tenex is recommended only for children ages 12 and up.	Hypnosis treatment, including session length and frequency, should be determined by a medical professional.
Active Ingredients	Guanfacine	N/A
Common Mild Side Effects	Dizziness, drowsiness, lightheadedness, dry mouth, constipation	None
Less Common Serious Side Effects	Allergic reaction, irregular heartbeat, pounding chest, decreased sexual function, changes in mood or behavior, fainting, blurred vision	None

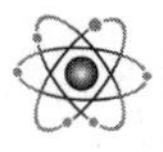

Science Says

The famous psychologist Milton Erickson first pioneered the use of hypnosis as a medical treatment for children. This work has continued over the years including a study by the Department of Pediatrics at Case Western Reserve University in Cleveland, Ohio. Researchers examined the practicality of self-hypnosis standardized methods in treating Tourette's syndrome patients with tics. In total, 79 percent of patients experienced a positive sustained clinical response over a six-week period. In fact, 46 percent achieved tic control through self-hypnosis after only two sessions, while 96 percent had success after three visits.

Natural Selection

Magnesium is essential for a healthy nervous system and can be found naturally in foods like soybeans, nuts, and whole grains. Other vitamins that improve nervous system functioning include vitamin B_6 and other B-complex vitamins. Chickpeas, bell peppers, and whole-grain breads are rich in these vitamins and can relax nervous system functioning, thereby reducing Tourette's syndrome symptoms. Finally, consider Ningdong granule, a Chinese herbal preparation that can regulate bodily production of dopamine to reduce the frequency and severity of Tourette's syndrome tics. Researchers at Shandong University in China demonstrated that Ningdong granule was safe and effective in an eight-week randomized, placebo-controlled, double-blind study in subjects ages 7 to 18 years with Tourette's syndrome.

Spotlight On: Acupuncture

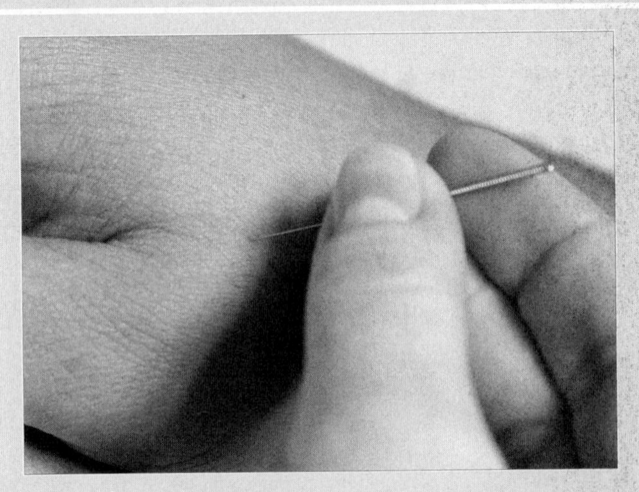

An acupuncture needle.

"Acupuncture is safe and is not a painful procedure. Children can easily accept acupuncture, particularly when it is demonstrated on a parent. One of the things children appreciate about it is that they can almost immediately feel its calming effects, so that even kids who are anxious about the procedure can relax. Children often get fast results in pain relief from acupuncture."

—Ellen Silver Highfield, Licensed Acupuncturist, Director of Acupuncture Programs and Assistant Professor of Family Medicine, Boston University School of Medicine

Originating in traditional Chinese medicine (TCM), the theory of acupuncture is based on a premise that bodily functions are regulated by energy flow (chi) in the body. The job of acupuncture is to correct energy flow imbalances by stimulating anatomical under-the-skin locations (referred to as acupuncture points) along pathways called meridians. Classically, these points are stimulated by tiny, hair-thin needles but also can be triggered by touch-pressure or heat.

According to TCM, the body has a delicate balance of two inseparable and opposing forces, yin and yang. Yin represents the slow and passive principle while yang represents the excited and active principle. Maintaining the body in a balanced state is critical for overall health. When imbalance occurs, acupuncture can unblock energy flow breakdowns and help restore the body to health.

Hundreds of studies have been conducted on the efficacy and safety of acupuncture for a host of ailments. For chronic pain especially, multiple trials have demonstrated the value of acupuncture. More specific to the ailments discussed in this chapter, researchers at Memorial Sloan-Kettering Cancer Center in New York City studied acupuncture in helping treat chronic headache disorders. Researchers discovered that acupuncture has persistent and clinically relevant benefits for patients experiencing chronic headaches, particularly migraines.

Your child may shiver at the thought of inserting a host of needles into her skin, yet studies have shown that acupuncture is well tolerated by children of all ages. There is a curious sensation when a needle is first inserted, one that feels to some like a single hair pulled on the skin. Then again, a small hair pull may be a small price to pay for easing the pain of persistent headaches.

13

Behavioral and Developmental Difficulties

"Increasing the consumption of omega-3 fats in foods or through supplementation, along with a balanced and healthy diet, has been shown to promote mental health in children. This is especially true for children with complex neurodevelopmental conditions like ADHD or autism. I take omega-3 supplements every single day and recommend them to every parent and child in my practice."

—Jay N. Gordon, MD, FAAP, Assistant Professor of Pediatrics, UCLA Medical School, www.drjaygordon.com

This is not a chapter about the common cold or easily handled childhood ailments. In this chapter, we're covering the heavy hitters, those behavioral and developmental difficulties that can be incurable and wreak havoc with a family's life.

That doesn't mean this chapter and its associated ailments are without hope. As you'll soon read, symptoms of even challenging conditions such as autism, bipolar disorder, and obsessive-compulsive disorder can be ameliorated by specific nutritional plans and supplements.

If your child has been diagnosed with one of the disorders covered in this chapter, rest assured you are not alone. Thousands of parents just like you have faced what lies ahead in these pages. So let's review both conventional remedies and treatment alternatives for behavioral and developmental conditions.

ADHD/ADD

Attention Deficit Hyperactive Disorder (ADHD) and Attention Deficit Disorder (ADD) are medical conditions associated with impulsivity, restlessnes, and difficulty concentrating. Originally, ADHD and ADD were considered separate disorders, but ADD is now commonly classified as ADHD without the hyperactivity component.

It is now estimated that nearly 10 percent of school-age children are diagnosed with some form of ADHD. Historically more boys than girls are diagnosed and the condition has a genetic component, though environmental triggers are clearly involved.

In very young children, symptoms of ADD and ADHD can be confused with typical childhood behavior—like running around aimlessly. In older children, common symptoms include short attention span, difficulty concentrating in class, sloppy schoolwork or chores at home, inability to sit still, and extreme disorganization.

While some children will outgrow ADD and ADHD symptoms naturally, treatment is often required for a child to realize his full academic (and eventually professional) potential. The following conventional remedies and treatment alternatives can help your child if he's dealing with ADD or ADHD.

ADHD/ADD Side-by-Side Comparison

	Conventional Remedy	Treatment Alternative
Generic Treatment	Methylphenidate	Neurofeedback
Sample Brand Name Treatment	Ritalin	N/A

	Conventional Remedy	Treatment Alternative
How it works	Ritalin manipulates chemicals in the brain that contribute to symptoms of ADHD/ADD such as impulsivity and hyperactivity.	During neurofeedback treatment, electrodes are applied to the skull and activity is recorded to determine periods during which the brain is focused. These brain waves are rewarded with positive feedback and imagery on the computer screen to which the electrodes are connected. Over time, the brain is conditioned to focus and concentrate because these brain patterns receive positive feedback.
Dosage	Dosage is determined by a doctor; common dose is between 10-60mg per day and is based on factors such as age and need. Tablets should be taken 30-45 minutes before a meal and early in the day to prevent sleep disturbances.	Neurotherapy should be performed only by a trained professional. Session length and frequency are determined by a professional and vary based upon the individual.
Active Ingredients	Methylphenidate	N/A
Common Mild Side Effects	Insomnia, nervousness, weight loss, nausea, vomiting, numbness or tingling, sweating, mild rash, dizziness, mild vision impairments, mild headache, decreased appetite, stomach pain	None

	Conventional Remedy	Treatment Alternative
Less Common Serious Side Effects	Allergic reaction, irregular heartbeat, lightheadedness, fever, twitching, shortness of breath, fever, headache, sore throat, blistering, peeling, rash, unusual behavior (aggression, restlessness, etc.), unexplained bruising, high blood pressure, anxiety, confusion, chest pain, seizure	None

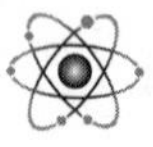

Science Says

Researchers at the Institute of Medical Psychology and Behavioral Neurology at Eberhard-Karls University in Germany compared neurofeedback versus methylphenidate in children with ADHD. In total, 34 children between the ages of 8 and 12 were assigned to the neurofeedback or methylphenidate group according to parental preference. Results showed both treatments led to equivalent improvements on all subscales of the Test of Variables of Attention. A second study at the University of Gottingen in Germany evaluated 102 children, ages 8 to 12, who performed either 36 sessions of neurofeedback training or a computerized attention skills training over a four-week period. For both parent and teacher ratings, improvements in the neurofeedback group were superior to those of the control group.

Natural Selection

Kathi J. Kemper, MD, MPH, Director of the Center for Integrative Medicine at Wake Forest University and author of *The Holistic Pediatrician* and *Mental Health, Naturally,* urges, "When it comes to ADHD and ADD, avoid artificial flavors, colors, and sweeteners. If it was made in nature, eat it; if it was genetically modified, ate something genetically modified, or was raised or made in a factory, don't."

Concentration can be improved and hyperactivity can be reduced with Pycnogenol extract. Originating from the bark of the French maritime pine tree, Pycnogenol is usually dosed starting at 50mg each morning. For the most natural approach to helping children with ADD/ADHD, look to nature itself. Research has shown there is a direct correlation between time spent outdoors at play and reduced ADD/ADHD symptoms.

Anger and Tantrums

Don't you just wish you could throw a temper tantrum at work? Your boss hands you a difficult assignment and you stomp around her office, tell her you hate her, and fall on the floor screaming at the top of your lungs. Wouldn't life be grand if that behavior didn't cost you your job? Well, kids often get away with anger and temper tantrums because we can't fire them!

Abrupt displays of frustration or rage characterize anger and temper tantrums. Screaming, crying, and flailing are some common traits of the inconsolable child. As your child grows, so does her understanding of the world. Unfortunately, childhood emotions don't always progress on the same timeline. Some of the most common reasons for an outburst include the following:

- Wanting to do something independently when a parent prefers to help
- Wanting a toy, game, or food treat and hearing the word *no* from a parent or caretaker
- Fatigue, hunger, thirst, illness, or other symptoms where a child simply feels "off"
- The inability to do something because of height, age, or other restrictions

Without the self-control, logic, and reasoning skills of an adult, anger and temper tantrums are a natural part of the maturation process. As the helpless parent experiencing a tantrum in line at the grocery store, you may want to learn about the remedy choices discussed here.

Anger and Tantrums Side-by-Side Comparison

	Conventional Remedy	Treatment Alternative
Generic Treatment	Time out	Free outdoor play
Sample Brand Name Treatment	1-2-3 Magic	N/A
How it works	1-2-3 Magic is a discipline technique used for the purpose of managing temper tantrums in children. With this method, three verbal warnings are given as needed for undesirable behavior associated with anger or tantrums. If a third warning is necessary, it is issued, along with a period of time out, the length of which is determined by the age of the child (one minute per year of age).	Free time outdoors will help provide children with a natural outlet for emotions such as anger and stress. The ability to run and play helps to boost positive endorphins. Time spent outdoors is thought to improve mood and concentration.
Dosage	Use as needed to help manage and reduce the incidence of temper tantrums.	Implement daily to help manage and reduce the incidence of temper tantrums.
Active Ingredients	N/A	N/A

	Conventional Remedy	Treatment Alternative
Common Mild Side Effects	None	None
Less Common Serious Side Effects	None	None

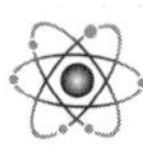

Science Says

School recess and group classroom behavior was analyzed by the Department of Pediatrics at Albert Einstein College of Medicine in New York City. The study analyzed the amount of recess for children ages 8 and 9 in the United States and its impact on behavior in the classroom. In total, more than 10,000 children were analyzed. Researchers determined that children experiencing at least one daily recess period of 15 minutes or longer achieved higher rating of class behavior scores by teachers.

Natural Selection

Communication with your child is critical in helping him deal with emotions and appropriate responses to them. Harvey Karp, MD, Creator of the *Happiest Toddler on the Block* DVD/book, offers this sage advice. "The key to success in quickly reducing a toddler's tantrums is to change your way of speaking to a more primitive, 3-step language, I call 'toddler-ese.' Sincerely acknowledging your child's feelings using short (1–4 word) phrases, repetition (4–10 times) and reflecting about ⅓ of your child's level of upset in your tone of voice and gestures can stop over 50% of tantrums … often in seconds."

Low blood sugar is thought to negatively impact childhood behavior by creating an adrenalin release that leads to behavior imbalances. A balanced diet is key, as well as a nutritious breakfast shortly after waking when children often have low energy from a night's sleep. Finally, omega-3 fatty acids are thought to promote solid sleeping habits and help reduce instances of negative childhood behavior.

Anxiety/Stress

It's hard to believe a 5-year-old can get stressed out. With no bills to pay, mortgage to cover, or long commute, what could possibly freak out a child? Then again, when the sandbox is your office, turf wars (or should we say sand wars) can break out at a moment's notice.

Anxiety and stress are emotions triggered by internal or external pressures placed on your child. These stressors can grow as he ages and may include bullying, unstable home life, routine disruption, and even too much schoolwork or too many activities.

✓ Good to Know

Thousands of years ago, the stress response was critical for survival. Our early ancestors needed a fight-or-flight response for nature's unexpected emergencies like wild animals attacking. Today's stressors are not typically life-threatening (e.g., a big test coming up), yet the body reacts in the same chemically induced way: muscles tense, breathing quickens, and the heart pounds. Chronic stress, the kind we experience most often these days, has a different chemical impact on the mind and body and is thought to be more harmful than acute stress.

When under stress, your child may exhibit a range of symptoms including bad habits (for example, nail biting), regression in school, bed-wetting (for younger children), insomnia, unstable emotions, withdrawal from friends and family, and anger. Physical ailments can even join the fray, including nausea, stomach pain, and fatigue.

If your child is acting like an accountant on April 14, you'll want to review the following conventional remedies and treatment alternatives available for consideration.

Anxiety/Stress Side-by-Side Comparison

	Conventional Remedy	Treatment Alternative
Generic Treatment	Diazepam	Yoga
Sample Brand Name Treatment	Valium	N/A
How it works	Valium is prescribed to provide relief from anxiety and stress. It works by manipulating the chemicals in the brain that cause feelings of anxiousness.	Yoga uses a combination of deep breathing, stretching, movement, and poses to reduce anxiety and stress. It can also inspire feelings of balance, relaxation, and focus.
Dosage	Not for use in children under 6 months of age; dosage is determined by a doctor. Common dose in children: 1-2mg per dose, taken 1-4 times per day	Certain styles of yoga are targeted toward stress reduction. These include Satyananda and Hatha yoga practices (but any yoga style may be helpful for building kids' stress-coping skills).
Active Ingredients	Diazepam	N/A
Common Mild Side Effects	Diarrhea, dizziness, upset stomach, change in appetite, fatigue, dry mouth, weakness, constipation, memory impairment, slurred speech, problems with vision, mild rash, or itching	None

	Conventional Remedy	Treatment Alternative
Less Common Serious Side Effects	Allergic reaction, seizure, tremor, restlessness, fever, yellowing of the skin or eyes, irregular heartbeat, changes in behavior (such as confusion, hallucinations, anger, or aggression), changes in urination or lack of bladder control, lightheadedness, shallow breathing	None

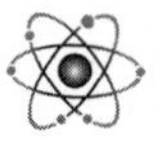

Science Says

Researchers at Flushing Hospital in Queens, New York, studied the effects of yoga on inner-city children's well-being. This pilot study compared fourth- and fifth-graders at two after-school programs in Bronx, New York. One offered an hourly yoga class for twelve weeks; the other did not. The yoga group reported using fewer negative behaviors when experiencing stress and had better balance than the control group.

Natural Selection

Valerian root is a natural anxiety-reducer. Pure Encapsulation makes a pleasant-tasting liquid form. When taken at bedtime, valerian can help ensure a restful night of sleep. You can also consider melatonin. This neurohormone helps normalize the body's ability to handle stress while maintaining proper sleep schedules. Finally, hypnosis can retrain the brain's thought processes and reasoning skills. Feelings of anxiety and stress can be reduced or eliminated when the mind is retrained to focus on calming thoughts.

Autism Spectrum Disorder

Autism Spectrum Disorder (ASD) is a whole-body neurodevelopmental disorder impacting a person's communication, behavioral, and social development. It's important to note in this section that the treatment alternatives discussed are for managing symptoms, not to truly cure the disorder.

Definitive causes of ASD are unknown but are thought to be related to the influence of various environmental factors in genetically predisposed children, predominantly males. There are different types of autism; in some cases, developmental delays are present from birth, while in others they first appear between one and three years of age. While no two cases are identical, frequent symptoms include the following:

- Repetitive movements such as rocking or arm-flapping
- Over- or under-reactions to external stimuli
- Lack of verbal development or verbal regression
- Sensitivity to sounds, scents, or touch
- Atypical eye contact when conversing

As children age, additional symptoms may include difficulty sharing, inability to maintain friendships, trouble displaying emotions, and an inability to perceive or display social cues. One or two of these symptoms is not typically an indicator of either disorder; this may simply be normal childhood behavior. The presence of quite a few of the symptoms interfering with daily functioning may point toward autism. It is very important to have your child evaluated promptly if you suspect one of these conditions. Early intervention can make a world of difference.

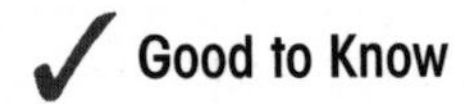

In the last 10 years alone, the prevalence rate of children diagnosed with Autism Spectrum Disorders has doubled to over 1 percent of children. While greater awareness of autism may explain some of the increase, many experts now agree that environmental factors play a significant role.

It's important to note that a high percentage of children with ASD experience gastrointestinal (GI) issues. Many treatment alternatives in this chapter are nutritionally-based for this reason.

Autism Spectrum Disorder Side-by-Side Comparison

	Conventional Remedy	Treatment Alternative
Generic Treatment	Risperidone	GFCF diet
Sample Brand Name Treatment	Risperdal	N/A
How it works	Risperdal is a prescription medicine used to help treat some symptoms of autism, such as aggression, rapid mood fluctuation, self-harm, and irritability.	With a gluten-free, casein-free diet, foods and beverages containing gluten and casein are eliminated from the diet in an effort to reduce symptoms of autism. Children with autism are thought to have problems digesting the proteins and peptides found in foods containing gluten and casein, which, according to theory, may exacerbate symptoms of autism.

	Conventional Remedy	Treatment Alternative
Dosage	Dosage is determined by a doctor. Oral tablets are available in 6 dosage strengths, which range from 0.25 to 4mg.	The removal of these items should be done only under the direction of a medical professional. It may be suggested that these are gradually removed from the diet in order to allow for a smoother transition for the body.
Active Ingredients	Risperidone	N/A
Common Mild Side Effects	Fatigue, dizziness, dry mouth, increased appetite, restlessness, upper respiratory tract infection, nausea, vomiting, rhinitis, coughing, bladder leakage, increased saliva, constipation, fever	Calcium deficiency, if dietary needs aren't met
Less Common Serious Side Effects	Allergic reaction, high fever, muscle stiffness, irregular heartbeat, diabetes, tremor, confusion, sweating, weakness, lightheadedness, high blood sugar, blood pressure problems, hyper-prolactinemia, Tardive Dyskinesia, seizures, involuntary movements, low white blood cell count, dizziness upon standing, suicidal thoughts, impaired judgment, infections,	None

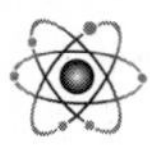

Science Says

At the Department of Pharmacy, Health and Well-Being at the University of Sunderland in the United Kingdom, researchers studied the effectiveness of a gluten-free, casein-free (GFCF) diet for children with ASD. In a 2-stage, 24-month, randomized, controlled trial, nearly 75 children, ages 4 to 11, were assigned to a GFCF diet or not. Those on the GFCF diet showed significant improvements in the Autism Diagnostic Observation Schedule (ADOS) and Gilliam Autism Rating Scale (GARS) compared to the control group. Results showed that dietary intervention may positively impact the developmental outcome for children diagnosed with autism spectrum disorders.

Natural Selection

Daily multivitamins can help reduce anger, aggression, and irritability in children with autism by addressing nutritional imbalances that may be leading to brain dysfunction. Similarly, an increase in omega-3 fatty acid consumption is believed to improve behavioral issues and motor skills while reducing hyperactivity. Finally, the Department of Psychiatry at Saint Francis Hospital in Hartford, Connecticut, demonstrated that a multimodal yoga, dance, and music therapy program significantly improved behavior, communication, and social skills in children with autism.

Bipolar Disorder/Mood Regulation

All children have mood swings. Some, though, have such incredible difficulty regulating their feelings so that they cannot function at home or at school. The most severe form of mood dysregulation, bipolar disorder, is characterized by extreme mood variations including periods of mania and/or periods of depression. The manic phase includes a range of symptoms such as excessive talking, hallucinations, lack of fatigue, grandiosity, and preoccupation with an idea or activity. Conversely, the depressive phase is characterized by withdrawal from friends, family, and daily activities; persistent sleeping or fatigue; extreme irritability; and feelings of hopelessness or worthlessness.

The most challenging part of parenting a child with bipolar disorder can be the rapid and unexpected swing in moods and behavior. A manic phase can quickly jump to a depressive state with little or no warning.

Prior to an official diagnosis of bipolar disorder, you may notice any of the following symptoms in your child:

- Severe irritability with little provocation
- Extreme aggression toward family or extreme separation anxiety for younger children
- Hearing or seeing things that are simply not there
- Impulsive actions with little or no regard for consequences

Similar to the discussion on autism spectrum disorders, the treatment alternatives covered here are not cures for bipolar disorder. However, they can help with mood regulation to minimize the severity of symptoms.

Bipolar Disorder/Mood Regulation Side-by-Side Comparison

	Conventional Remedy	Treatment Alternative
Generic Treatment	Aripiprazole	Vitamins & minerals
Sample Brand Name Treatment	Abilify	EMPower Plus

	Conventional Remedy	Treatment Alternative
How it works	Alters chemicals in the brain that contribute to the way the brain processes and reacts to information	EMPower Plus tablets are a nutritional supplement containing vitamins, minerals, amino acids, and antioxidants that help resolve nutritional deficiencies and may significantly reduce symptoms of bipolar disorder.
Dosage	Dosage is determined by a doctor. Abilify is used in children ages 10 to 17. It is taken once daily with or without food.	Consult a doctor before use. Suggested use is 4 tablets twice daily with food.
Active Ingredients	Aripiprazole	Vitamins A, B_6, B_{12}, C, D, E, thiamin, riboflavin, niacin, folic acid, biotin, pantothenic acid, calcium, iron, phosphorus, iodine, magnesium, zinc, selenium, copper, manganese, chromium, molybdenum, potassium
Common Mild Side Effects	Drowsiness, dizziness, restlessness, nausea, blurred vision, weight gain, drooling, tremor	Gastrointestinal upset
Less Common Serious Side Effects	Allergic reaction, diabetes, hyperglycemia, suicidal thoughts, unusual change in behavior, new or worsened mood symptoms, stroke, high fever, irregular heartbeat, severe tremor, sweating, confusion, Tardive Dyskinesia	None (if taken properly and as directed by a doctor; possible iron overdose if taken improperly)

Science Says

At the University of Canterbury in New Zealand, researchers examined the effects of children with bipolar disorder consuming a 36-ingredient micronutrient formula (EMPower Plus). In total, 120 children were studied in 11 different trials. The mean symptom severity of reported bipolar symptoms was 46 percent lower than baseline in these open-label trials. The growing body of research from these studies strongly suggests that micronutrients show a therapeutic benefit for children with bipolar disorder. Given the paucity of observed side effects compared to conventional treatments, the opportunity exists for a reduction in the psychiatric medications while still improving ailment symptoms.

Natural Selection

Similar to previous ailments covered in this chapter, omega-3 fatty acids can help promote mood stabilization. Additionally, healthy nutrition, consistent sleep patterns, and regular exercise help regulate moods. Exercise in particular releases endorphins, which help to modulate hostile and aggressive emotions.

Depression

Feeling blue accompanies even the happiest childhood—it's the persistent presence of sadness that indicates depression. It's unrelenting and can interfere with daily functioning at home, in school, and with friends.

While no single cause of depression is known, it can be attributed to a number of factors including environmental issues, physical or emotional health, and life events (e.g., a difficult illness or death in the family). Depression also has genetic links as depressed children often have a family history of the condition.

The most common signs of depression include lack of energy, fatigue, friend/family withdrawal, frequent crying, persistent sadness, extreme irritability, and feelings of worthlessness or hopelessness. As children get older, these symptoms may be accompanied by substance abuse, reckless sexual behavior, and morbid or suicidal thoughts.

When symptoms persist for longer than two or three weeks, it's worth investigating to see if it's a case of depression. While a strong family and friend support system is most important in handling depression, these conventional remedies and treatment alternatives can also offer some relief.

Depression Side-by-Side Comparison

	Conventional Remedy	Treatment Alternative
Generic Treatment	Fluoxetine	Omega-3 fatty acids
Sample Brand Name Treatment	Prozac	Nordic Naturals ProOmega Junior
How it works	Prozac is a prescription medication that is used to treat depression. It affects the chemical serotonin and the way the brain processes messages.	Nordic Naturals ProOmega Junior is an omega-3 supplement for children that provides support for healthy brain function.
Dosage	Take only as prescribed by a doctor. Prozac may be taken with or without food. Common pediatric dose is 10-20mg per day. It is typically prescribed only for adults and children over the age of 7.	Take 2 softgels per day or as recommended by a medical professional; 2 softgels contain 640mg total omega-3s (325mg EPA and 225mg DHA)
Active Ingredients	Fluoxetine hydrochloride	Omega-3

	Conventional Remedy	Treatment Alternative
Common Mild Side Effects	Drowsiness, unusual dreams, flu-like symptoms, diarrhea, sexual problems, loss of appetite, change in sleeping habits, minor tremor, yawning, sinus infection, fatigue, minor sweating, mild rash, anxiety or nervousness, increased thirst, nosebleed, frequent urination, hot flashes, heavy menstrual periods, slower growth rate, abnormal increase in muscle movement, dry mouth, constipation	None
Less Common Serious Side Effects	Allergic reaction, suicidal thoughts or actions, acting on dangerous impulses, behaving aggressively or violently, new or worsened depression, difficulty sleeping, new or worsened panic attacks, agitation or restlessness, abnormal increase in talking or activity, unusual change in mood or behavior, hallucinations, coma or abnormal changes in mental status, irregular heartbeat, nausea, vomiting, low or high blood pressure, muscle rigidity, changes in weight, headache, weakness, sweating, fever, confusion, issues with coordination, great increase in energy, racing thoughts, reckless behavior, grandiose ideas, excessive happiness or irritability, memory problems, muscle spasms, loss of consciousness	Allergic reaction

Natural Selection

As with bipolar disorders, a key to coping with depression includes focusing on good nutrition, sleep, and exercise. As Timothy Culbert, MD, FAAP, further indicates:

> "Sedentary lifestyles can contribute to depression. I suggest more time in nature and 'earthing' practices. Redesigning academic, social, and home environments so kids experience more consistent positive feedback, social connections, and recognition of their strengths and talents as a person are all important changes as well."

Studies also specifically suggest that certain B vitamins like folate are found in lower amounts in depressed children. Natural light and light therapy, perhaps involving vitamin D mechanisms, can also help alleviate depression symptoms. Finally, yoga is one of several mind-body therapies that can act as a mood-lifter.

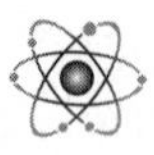

Science Says

At the Department of Psychiatry at the University of Cincinnati, researchers investigated the connection between omega-3 fatty acid deficiencies and mood disorders. Omega-3 fatty acid deficiency is associated with mood disorders and dietary omega-3 supplementation is well tolerated and effectively corrects these deficiencies. Omega-3 supplementation adds to the efficacy of medications in the treatment of mood symptoms and may in fact be effective as a solo treatment for mood disorders in children and adolescents.

Night Terrors

"Daddy, daddy, I just had a terrible dream that Elmo stopped sharing and grabbed my Hot Wheels race car without asking. Can I sleep in bed with you and mommy tonight?" Whether you let your little one co-sleep or coddle them back into bed is your decision. Either way, this is not a case of night terrors, just a bad dream.

Night terrors are much more disruptive and include a number of characteristics, including screaming while asleep, sleepwalking, thrashing in bed, and persistent sweating or rapid heartbeat. Also, children experiencing night terrors typically have zero recollection of the experience. In contrast, your child can usually recall a nightmare the next day.

While night terrors can occur at any age, the most common range is preschool through elementary school. In most cases, children will outgrow night terrors, although the condition can be exacerbated by stress, anxiety, illness, new medications, or sleep deprivation. Check out these treatment alternatives to keep night terrors at bay.

Night Terrors Side-by-Side Comparison

	Conventional Remedy	Treatment Alternative
Generic Treatment	Observation	Ferrous gluconate
Sample Brand Name Treatment	N/A	Floradix Iron + Herbs
How it works	In an effort to monitor children who experience night terrors, it may be necessary to observe a child at home or in a sleep lab. This can help determine if there is a pattern. Observing night terrors can also ensure that the child does not sleepwalk or cause harm to him or herself.	Floradix Iron + Herbs provides proper amounts of iron without unpleasant side effects. It is kosher and suitable for vegetarians. An iron deficiency may be to blame for night terrors and Floradix will help to address the deficiency.

	Conventional Remedy	Treatment Alternative
Dosage	Children may be observed as needed by baby monitor, video monitor, in same room or sleep lab	Children 4-11: take 2 tsp once per day with food; children 12 years old and older: take 2 tsp twice daily with food.
Active Ingredients	N/A	Ferrous gluconate
Common Mild Side Effects	None	None
Less Common Serious Side Effects	None	None

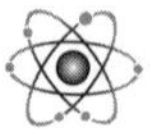

Science Says

Addressing mineral deficiencies may be effective for a variety of sleep disorders, including night terrors. At the Department of Nutritional Sciences at Penn State University in Pennsylvania, researchers studied the effects of iron and/or zinc supplementation on infant sleep patterns. In total, over 1,300 infants received iron-folic acid with or without zinc daily for 12 months with assessments conducted every 3 months. Maternal reports of sleep patterns were studied, including napping frequency and duration and frequency of night waking. Researchers discovered that micronutrient supplementation for infants at high risk for iron deficiency or iron deficiency anemia was connected to increased night sleep duration and less night waking.

Natural Selection

Zinc deficiency, as referenced, may contribute to night terrors. L-5-hydroxytryptophan (L-5-HTP) may also help to reduce or eliminate instances of night terrors. It can be taken in supplement form. Before giving zinc and L-5-HTP to your child, a medical professional should be consulted for exact dosage. Finally, consider hypnosis for a child with sleep concerns. Research has shown that hypnosis can retrain the body to fall asleep gradually rather than immediately drifting into deep sleep. This gradual process is thought to reduce the occurrence of night terrors.

Obsessive-Compulsive Disorder

Characterized by an involuntary preoccupation with illogical thoughts and fears, obsessive-compulsive disorder (OCD) causes a child to perform repetitive behaviors that interfere with daily living. Even when the repetitive behavior is not performed, children have lingering or even debilitating worry about the task.

While the exact cause of OCD is unknown, it is thought to be linked to disruption of serotonin levels in the brain that impact normal thought processing. Obsessive and compulsive behaviors differ from each other. Examples of obsessive behaviors include the following:

- The desire to keep things in order or symmetrical
- Fears of dirt, grime, germs, or contamination
- Persistent fear of personal or familial harm or illness
- Obsession with a particular idea or object

Compulsive behaviors are more about repetitive behaviors. These may include brushing one's hair over and over again, repeatedly checking that doors or windows are locked, counting something relentlessly, or walking an identical route over and over.

Changes to a daily routine can trigger or exacerbate OCD symptoms. These may include rearranging furniture, moving to a new home, or changing schools. Additionally, as we noted in Chapter 12's discussion of Tourette's syndrome and tics, certain infections (like strep throat) can trigger acute-onset OCD symptoms—often associated with motor tics—also known as PANDAS. From medications to behavioral therapy, these treatment alternatives may help your child.

Obsessive Compulsive Disorder Side-by-Side Comparison

	Conventional Remedy	Treatment Alternative
Generic Treatment	Sertraline	Cognitive behavioral therapy
Sample Brand Name Treatment	Zoloft	N/A
How it works	Zoloft is part of a group of drugs called selective serotonin reuptake inhibitors, (SSRIs) which help the brain transmit and receive messages while also helping to restore the balance of serotonin in the brain, thereby reducing the symptoms of OCD.	Cognitive behavioral therapy is a form of psychotherapy that emphasizes awareness and regaining control over one's thoughts and behaviors. It is an active therapy with a focus on goals and making progress toward these goals.
Dosage	Dosage is determined by a medical professional, though a common dosage in children ages 6-12 is 25mg per day. A common dosage for children ages 13-17 is 50mg per day.	Cognitive behavioral therapy should be conducted as recommended by a medical professional.
Active Ingredients	Sertraline hydrochloride	N/A
Common Mild Side Effects	Drowsiness, fever, loss of bladder control, nosebleed, red or purple skin discoloration, aggression, sinus infection, acne, hyperactivity	None

	Conventional Remedy	Treatment Alternative
Less Common Serious Side Effects	Allergic reaction, agitation, hallucinations, coma or change in mental condition, irregular heartbeat, coordination issues or muscle spasms, high or low blood pressure, nausea, diarrhea, vomiting, muscle stiffness or tightness, headache, unusual bleeding or bruising, weakness, loss of balance, confusion, trouble thinking or focusing, memory problems, suicidal thoughts or behavior, anxiety, panic attacks, high fever, weight gain, hair loss	None

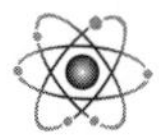

Science Says

At the UCLA-Semel Institute for Neuroscience and Human Behavior, scientists examined cognitive-behavioral therapy (CBT) for treating OCD in children and adolescents. Authors noted that CBT is "now widely recognized as the gold standard intervention for childhood OCD." Relying on exposure and response prevention, CBT has been demonstrated to be equally effective to SSRI medications like sertraline for pediatric OCD.

Natural Selection

In one small, controlled trial, *Silybum marianum* (more commonly known as milk thistle) was found to be just as effective as fluoxetine (Prozac) for OCD. Dietary supplements inositol and N-acetyl cysteine may be effective in some cases of OCD; both have been studied in cases of treatment-resistant patients. Additionally, kundalini yoga, acupuncture, and mindfulness meditation all have some data to suggest they can alleviate symptoms of OCD.

Sleep Problems

Have you ever put your toddler to sleep at 7 P.M. and marveled that they slept until 7 A.M. the next morning? What you wouldn't give for a twelve-spot! You may not even get that in two nights combined.

It's recommended that growing children get at least 10 hours of sleep per night. Unfortunately, many children fall short due to sleep problems and sleep deprivation. As parents know, a lack of sleep can influence mood, behavior, and performance in school. Of course, parents expect night wakings for newborns and even younger toddlers, but when the problem persists beyond early years you likely have a sleep problem that requires further attention.

The most common symptoms of sleep problems include an inability to fall asleep within 30 minutes, multiple night wakings, trouble waking in the morning, and daytime fatigue. In some cases, these issues can be easily resolved through daily routine or environmental changes (i.e., eating dinner further away from bedtime or changing the nighttime thermostat). Unfortunately, there's not always an easier answer, and you'll need to investigate these treatment alternatives.

Sleep Problems Side-by-Side Comparison

	Conventional Remedy	Treatment Alternative
Generic Treatment	Clonidine	Melatonin
Sample Brand Name Treatment	Catapres	Pure Encapsulations Melatonin

	Conventional Remedy	Treatment Alternative
How it works	Catapres can help resolve sleep problems by lowering heart rate and relaxing blood vessels, which has a calming effect on children and allows them to doze off to sleep more easily.	Pure Encapsulations Melatonin is a hormonal supplement that helps to regulate the body's natural sleep cycle based upon periods of daylight and darkness.
Dosage	Dosage is determined by a medical professional and is determined by a child's weight. Common dosage in children is 0.1-0.2mg per day.	Dosage varies from 0.5-3mg per day. Proper usage and dosage in children should be determined by a doctor. Capsule should be taken 30-60 minutes before bedtime.
Active Ingredients	Clonidine hydrochloride	Melatonin
Common Mild Side Effects	Dizziness, dry mouth, constipation, mild sedation, drowsiness, blurred vision, nausea, vomiting, headache, muscle or joint pain, mild rash, insomnia, lightheadedness	Daytime drowsiness (for bedtime use only)
Less Common Serious Side Effects	Allergic reaction, edema, weakness, congestive heart failure, hypotension, bradycardia, increased heart rate, heart rate of less than 60 beats per minute, shortness of breath, fever, paleness, decreased urination, swelling, weight gain	None

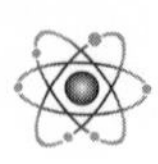

Science Says

At the Department of Neurology and Sleep-Wake Disorders in The Netherlands, researchers studied melatonin as a treatment for chronic sleep onset insomnia in children. In the study, 40 elementary school children ages 6 to 12 were examined. Each participant had suffered at least one year of chronic insomnia. The children received either 5 milligrams of melatonin or a placebo. After four months of trial, researchers found that melatonin was significantly more effective than a placebo in advancing sleep onset and increasing sleep duration.

Natural Selection

Lavender aromatherapy can help promote relaxation and lead to an easier time falling asleep. Place five drops of lavender essential oil in a small spray bottle filled with water. Shake well and then spray onto a pillow before bedtime. Guided imagery can help a child both fall asleep faster and stay asleep longer. Conducted by a medical professional or with a CD, your child's thoughts will be directed toward relaxation, peace, and sleep. For babies, white noise sound machines have been known to simulate the sounds of a mother's womb, thereby helping babies fall asleep and stay asleep longer.

Speech Development/Stuttering

Stuttering interferes with normal speech development patterns and is characterized by long silences, partial sound repetition, or the drawing out of syllables. Any of these speech conditions negatively affect the normal fluency of speech. Children suffering from stuttering or other speech problems often feel frustrated or angry by their inability to communicate clearly. Worse yet, in older kids, being made fun of or bullied at school only worsens negative feelings.

Stuttering is one common speech problem, but others include the following:

- Dyspraxia: impaired ability of the tongue, lips, and mouth to synchronize properly in vocalizing sounds and words
- Dysarthria: a nervous system disorder that slows or slurs speech due to a weakness or paralysis of the face or mouth
- Orofacial myofunctional disorder: a muscular disorder where the tongue moves too far forward in the mouth and affects the pronunciation of certain sounds or syllables

Speech therapy is a time-tested conventional treatment course for any of these speech development issues. Jan Klein, MA, CCC-SLP, points out, "If a speech-language disorder or delay is suspected, early detection, assessment, and intervention can be instrumental. Aside from remediation of the disorder and or delay itself, often the child's frustration level is reduced, self-confidence is gained, and the family becomes educated on how to best help their child. Typically, session frequency and duration for speech therapy depend upon the nature and severity of the disorder and or delay." Often used in combination with speech therapy, nutritional supplements have been shown to add value for speech disorders.

Speech Development/Stuttering Side-by-Side Comparison

	Conventional Remedy	Treatment Alternative
Generic Treatment	Speech therapy	Omega 3, vitamin E, vitamin K
Sample Brand Name Treatment	N/A	Nourishlife SPEAK Capsules

	Conventional Remedy	Treatment Alternative
How it works	Speech therapy, which is performed by a speech pathologist, can help encourage speech development in areas where professional help may be needed, such as stuttering. This is done by first evaluating a child's speech, oral skills, feeding and swallowing abilities, and cognitive development. Next, an individualized course of treatment is determined.	SPEAK uses a special combination of vitamins and minerals to help promote healthy speech and coordination development in children experiencing problems in these areas. SPEAK also promotes neurological health.
Dosage	Duration and frequency of speech therapy is determined by a professional. Common areas of focus and therapy include articulation, phonetics, language, and cognitive development.	During the first two weeks, child should take 1 softgel daily; during weeks 3 and 4, take 2 softgels daily; during weeks 5 and 6, take 3 softgels daily; during weeks 7 and 8, take 4 softgels daily; during weeks 9 and 10, take 5 softgels daily; during weeks 11 and 12, take 6 softgels daily. Discuss with a healthcare professional before exceeding 4 capsules per day. Take in the morning and in the afternoon with food.

	Conventional Remedy	Treatment Alternative
Active Ingredients	N/A	Omega-3, vitamin E, vitamin K, GHA
Common Mild Side Effects	None	Temporary irritability, moodiness, emotional outbursts, diarrhea
Less Common Serious Side Effects	None	None

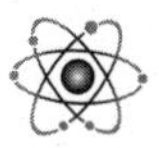

Science Says

The Children's Hospital and Research Center in Oakland, California, studied verbal apraxia, a neurologically based speech disorder common in autism spectrum disorders. The goal of this pilot study was to see how this condition responded to omega-3 and vitamin E supplementation. In total, 187 children were treated with vitamin E and polyunsaturated fatty acid supplementation. Over 97 percent of participating families reported dramatic improvements in a number of areas, including speech, eye contact, and sensory issues.

Natural Selection

Other nutritional supplements may promote a child's speech and language ability, as a complement to speech therapy. Methyl-B_{12} and folinic acid have been studied in autistic children with promising results. Finally, hypnosis is thought to help reduce or eliminate stuttering in children by assisting cognitive speech processes. As the child gets older, self-hypnosis can become a successful and easy-to-follow game plan for reducing stuttering.

Spotlight On: Kids Yoga

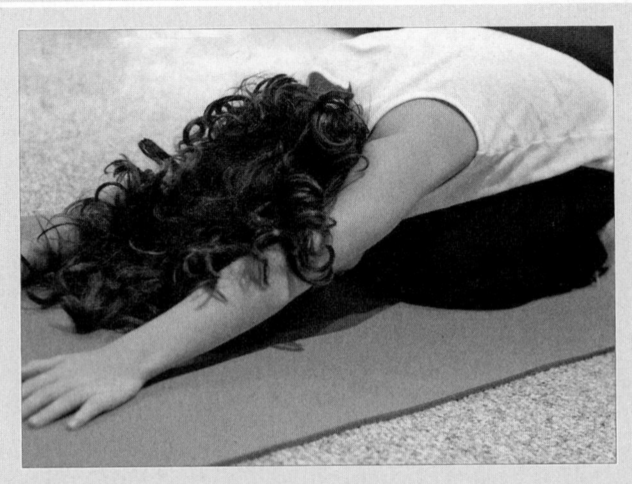

A child performing a yoga pose.

"Every day our children are inundated with stressful stimulation. Through the use of breath and guided meditation, children learn to quiet their minds and understand that they have the personal resources to self-soothe. The practice of yoga offers a road map to inner peace, centeredness, and self confidence."

—Geri Topfer (Founder and President) and Penny Feiner (Executive Director), Kula for Karma (www.kulaforkarma.org)

Before you dismiss the camel pose and downward dog as crazy animal gestures, researchers at the University of Mississippi Center for Health Behavior Research explored the therapeutic effects of yoga on improving quality of life. Examining published articles and research initiatives on yoga, they noted the multitude of ailments and conditions that can benefit therapeutically from yoga. Results showed that yoga enhances muscular strength and body flexibility while promoting improved cardiovascular and respiratory functioning. It can also reduce stress, anxiety, chronic pain, and sleep difficulties.

As an adult, you may associate yoga with challenging poses or extreme heat sessions. This is not what kids' yoga is all about. Instead, the goal is for children to begin exploring body movements that build flexibility, resilience, and strength, combined with learning calming breathing techniques and stress-relieving thought processes. In today's busy, overscheduled world, yoga may be the perfect antidote. Developing more relaxed, gentle, and optimistic-minded kids sure is a worthwhile goal for your family.

A

Toxic Troubles

If you just read this book cover to cover, you're officially an ailment and treatment alternative expert. Then again, maybe you decided to dive in and jump to the most relevant and timely ailments for your child.

Either way, you'll note that we focused on treating common conditions to give you practical tools to help your kids. However, we think prevention is so important to promoting children's health that we've included this appendix on environmental issues.

When you think about childhood ailments, you likely picture germs changing hands at toddlers' play dates or that coughing kid in fifth grade who should have stayed home from school. Diseases, though, are not simply a human-to-human infection phenomenon. There are a host of environmental threats to children's health that can lead to serious conditions such as asthma, cancer, and neurological issues.

This is not a call to keep your kids in the house until high school graduation. View this appendix as a precautionary tale on preventing the most common environmental exposures. After all, prevention is more effective than treatment when it comes to toxins like heavy metals and pesticides. Then again, there are some natural remedies (predominantly nutritional, though some are herbal) that can help to both prevent and remediate damage done by toxins.

Heavy Metals

Not to be confused with distorted guitars and big-hair shrieking, heavy metals in this section refer to toxic elements that cause harm to the environment and to people. The most common examples include arsenic, lead, and mercury. Heavy metal poisoning occurs when one of these elements is ingested, inhaled, or absorbed in large amounts —or in small amounts over a long period of time. The most common sources of exposure are from industrial pollution and can include the following:

- Arsenic: contaminated water, paints, hazardous waste sites
- Lead: paint, batteries, pesticides
- Mercury: fish, medical equipment (old thermometers or blood pressure devices), biological preservatives (thimerosal)

Symptoms vary depending on the heavy metal exposure and on the individual's ability to excrete the toxin (detoxification). Some of the most common symptoms of heavy metal poisoning include: headache, confusion, visual impairment, fatigue, nausea, vomiting, and changes in skin pigmentation. Heavy metal toxicity is most serious for pregnant women, women who are breastfeeding, and infants and children.

In dealing with heavy metal toxicity, a number of treatments have been researched and found to be potentially effective. Remember, though: prevention is always preferred to treatment when it comes to environmental exposures.

- Chelation therapy: This is the process of cleansing the body of damaging heavy metals and is done through the use of DMSA (dimercaptosuccinic acid), DMPS (2,3-dimercapto-1-propanesulfonic acid) and EDTA (ethylenediaminetetraacetic acid), typically administered orally or intravenously. These agents bind to the metals and help the body excrete them more quickly and efficiently than would typically be expected. Note, though, that chelation is a serious medical procedure with the potential for major adverse reactions and should only be used under the supervision of an experienced clinician. There are also gentler and natural forms of chelation to consider, particularly from foods such as garlic and cilantro.

- Ascorbic acid (vitamin C): may reduce brain and cellular damage associated with toxicity of lead
- N-acetyl cysteine, zinc, and selenium: a combination of all three may reverse damage caused by mercury exposure
- Melatonin: may reduce toxicity from exposure to high levels of arsenic

Sources:
www.ncbi.nlm.nih.gov/pubmed/17959157
www.ncbi.nlm.nih.gov/pubmed/22056337
www.ncbi.nlm.nih.gov/pubmed/21424224
www.ncbi.nlm.nih.gov/pubmed/15664430

Endocrine Disruptors

Synthetic chemicals that interfere with the functioning of the body's hormones are considered endocrine disruptors. Some of these chemicals actually change the way the body produces hormones like estrogen and testosterone, thereby damaging an otherwise healthy endocrine system. These exposures can lead to early or delayed puberty, impaired fertility, or certain cancers.

Examples of endocrine disruptors include agricultural chemicals (such as diethylstilbesterol or DES), pesticides (such as dichlorodiphenyl-trichloroethane or DDT), and herbicides. They can also be found in detergents, cosmetics, and plastics (like phthalates and bisphenol A or BPA). Fetal exposure to BPA and other plasticizers is particularly dangerous. This explains why some states and countries are banning its use, and manufacturers are finally removing it from baby bottles and other products.

Avoidance of these chemicals is the first crucial step. Interestingly, there are some natural remedies that may help protect us from the damage from these exposures. Specific probiotics such as *Bifidobacterium breve* strain Yakult (BbY) and *Lactobacillus casei* strain Shirota (LcS), have been shown to protect the body from absorbing BPA. Broccoli, cauliflower, and other organic cruciferous vegetables contain indole-3-carbynol compounds that promote the body's ability to rid itself of endocrine disruptors.

Sources:
www.epa.gov/endo/pubs/edspoverview/whatare.htm
www.nrdc.org/health/effects/qendoc.asp
www.ncbi.nlm.nih.gov/pubmed?term=bpa%20probiotics

Pesticides

Pesticides are chemicals typically used to protect produce and crops from pests such as bugs, insects, birds, rodents, and weeds. Unfortunately, human exposure to pesticides can cause health problems ranging from minor (e.g., skin irritation) to major (e.g., asthma, cancer, and neurological problems).

Beyond just crop protection, pesticides are also found in many bug and insect repellants. DEET (N,N-diethyl-m-toluamide) is applied topically to protect the human body from insects or bugs that may bite, sting, or carry diseases. It also has the potential to cause health problems from skin rashes to severe issues like neurological and neuromuscular disorders (including paralysis and trouble breathing). Permethrins, members of the pyrethroid class of pesticides, are the active ingredient in most over-the-counter lice treatments and may cause neurological toxicity at high doses.

The best way to reduce or eliminate kids' pesticide exposure is to choose pesticide-free home, garden, and cleaning products and organic fruits and vegetables when possible—these are grown without pesticides. The microbes found in probiotics may help reduce pesticide toxicity by binding to the chemicals to make them more easily excretable.

Sources:
www.epa.gov/pesticides/health/children-live.html
www.ncbi.nlm.nih.gov/pubmed/15952424

Air Pollution

Carbon monoxide, carbon dioxide, sulfur oxide, and nitrogen oxide are all examples of air pollution that can impact the atmosphere. Breathing these pollutants can pose a risk to both humans and animals. A range of sources cause air pollution, including aerosol deodorants and hairspray, smoke stacks, and transportation sources (like buses, cars, and boats). Direct exposures affect breathing, but of equal concern is the affect of air pollution on pregnant women and their babies. Air pollution exposure in these cases can lead to premature labor and neurological problems for the unborn child.

The risk from exposure to air pollution can be reduced in a number of ways, including:

- Choosing transportation methods that do not emit harmful gases
- Utilizing recyclable and renewable forms of energy
- Properly ventilating living spaces to prevent respiratory problems from pollutants

Maintaining healthy antioxidant and nutrient levels through intake of organic fruits and vegetables may also help limit the ill effects of air pollution.

Sources:
yosemite.epa.gov/ochp/ochpweb.nsf/content/outdoor_air_pollution.htm
www.ncbi.nlm.nih.gov/pubmed/21868304

Tobacco Smoke

Cigarettes and cigars are the biggest culprits when it comes to tobacco smoke. The numerous chemicals found in tobacco smoke are easily absorbed by the lungs. The chemicals also affect the cardiovascular and nervous systems. It has been known for a number of years that smoking tobacco can lead to a variety of cancers, respiratory problems, heart attacks, stroke, and emphysema.

For children the bigger risk is secondhand smoke. The toxic chemicals exhaled by smokers can actually cause more health problems than those experienced by the person smoking. For children, this can lead to asthma, bronchitis, ear infections, or pneumonia. It is also thought to increase the risk of sudden infant death syndrome in babies. Pregnant women exposed to secondhand smoke are at risk of premature birth, stillbirth, and low birth weight. More recently, data has clearly shown the negative effects of third-hand smoke—that is, the effect on infants and children (including those in utero) via tobacco smoke contamination that remains after the cigarette has been extinguished.

Besides avoiding exposures to environmental tobacco smoke, loading up on docosahexaenoic acid (DHA) has been found to reduce the risk of lung disease following smoke inhalation. DHA is an omega-3 fatty acid found in eggs, fish oils, nuts, and flax seeds. Also, turmeric and green tea extracts have a detoxifying effect that can protect the body from the harmful chemicals found in cigarette smoke.

Sources:

www.cdc.gov/tobacco/data_statistics/fact_sheets/secondhand_smoke/general_facts/index.htm
www.cancer.org/Cancer/CancerCauses/TobaccoCancer/secondhand-smoke
www.nytimes.com/2009/01/03/health/research/03smoke.html
www.ncbi.nlm.nih.gov/pubmed/10351918
www.ncbi.nlm.nih.gov/pubmed/15149152

Climate Change

Marked variations in weather patterns describe climate change. It's responsible for extreme temperature changes (like mild winters), floods, droughts, and hurricanes. While much of climate change is a natural occurrence, some is manmade from irreversible changes to the planet's climate caused by pollution, deforestation, and carbon dioxide. Global climate change clearly affects the environment and only now are we recognizing the major impact it has on human health.

Climate changes affect our health by affecting food supply—both crops and livestock. It also increases pollution, thereby affecting air quality and leading to respiratory problems, particularly in young children.

Climate change will also alter the areas in which insects can live and thrive. This poses a problem in that insects that carry diseases will be more easily spread throughout the world. Pollens and molds also thrive in warmer temperatures.

Changes in the earth's ozone layer lead to health problems in several ways. Breathing increased ozone is associated with respiratory problems like asthma. An increase in warmer weather means more exposure to harmful ultraviolet light. Studies also suggest that children who live in areas with known problems with air pollution are at risk of vitamin D deficiency and could therefore benefit from taking a vitamin D supplement. Vitamin D, in fact, may be protective against a number of climate change–related health effects.

Additionally, just as with many other environmental exposures, improving antioxidant status is helpful to limiting toxic damage. Glutathione, one of the body's main natural antioxidants, depends on adequate production of compounds like n-acetylcysteine (NAC). Ingesting NAC supplements may increase levels of glutathione. Healthy levels of glutathione are associated with improved immune and detoxification functions.

Sources:
www.epa.gov/climatechange/downloads/Climate_Change_Health.pdf
www.epa.gov/glo/health.html
www.ncbi.nlm.nih.gov/pubmed/12138058
www.ncbi.nlm.nih.gov/pubmed/18628525
www.ncbi.nlm.nih.gov/pubmed/21986034
www.ncbi.nlm.nih.gov/pubmed/21412082

Radiation

While exposure to high levels of radiation can have devastating effects on one's health, so can low levels of radiation when one is exposed over a period of time. Radiation exposure occurs through gamma rays, X-rays, UV rays, infrared rays, microwaves, and radio waves.

Ionizing radiation, the type that is high in frequency, has the potential to cause damage to human DNA and has carcinogenic properties. Ionizing radiation is found in gamma rays, X-rays, and some UV rays. Types of cancer associated with ionizing radiation include breast, lung, skin, and thyroid cancers.

Though levels of radiation are relatively low in single X-rays, cumulative or sporadic high-dose exposure (via CT scans, for example) may endanger the growing bodies of young children. Radiation can also cause birth defects in growing fetuses.

Exposure to high levels of radiation (specifically the iodine isotope 131I) through catastrophic disaster exposure causes a major increase in the risk of developing thyroid cancer. Potassium iodide can greatly reduce the risk of developing thyroid cancer following exposure to radiation.

Allylmethylsulfide (AMS), a derivative of garlic, serves as a radio-protective agent, helping to protect the body from the potentially devastating effects of radiation. Eating garlic is also thought to reduce the risk of developing skin cancer as a result of UV exposure.

Sources:
www.ncbi.nlm.nih.gov/pubmed/15900042
www.ncbi.nlm.nih.gov/pubmed/19627202
www.nlm.nih.gov/medlineplus/radiationexposure.html

Electromagnetic Fields (EMF)

Electromagnetic fields (EMF) are fields of energy that result from the use of electrical devices. Cell phones are a common example and research is inconclusive thus far on the long-term dangers of prolonged usage. There are concerns raised by heat and EMF exposure to the brain through the thin area of the skull near the ear.

Extract from *Silybum marianum,* better known as milk thistle, may serve as a protective agent in cases of EMF exposure. When used in extract form, astragalus—an herb commonly used in traditional Chinese medicine—can also help protect the body against radiation damage.

Sources:
www.cancer.org/Cancer/CancerCauses/OtherCarcinogens/MedicalTreatments/radiation-exposure-and-cancer
www.nlm.nih.gov/medlineplus/electromagneticfields.html
www.ncbi.nlm.nih.gov/pubmed/20653235
www.ncbi.nlm.nih.gov/pubmed/21075176

B

Top Ten Treatment Lists

You would not believe how many ailments can be treated without ever leaving your house. From the spice rack to common ingredients and garden-variety plants and herbs, you can treat and cure many ailments without trips to the drugstore. There's also a host of oils and homeopathics covered in this appendix that are readily available at your local natural store or online. Get ready to be amazed by what cranberry and garlic (and a host of other common ingredients and products) can do for your child.

Ten Spice Rack Resources

1. Basil

Basil is an herb that is also a natural expectorant. It is helpful in treating illnesses that involve excess mucus, such as a cold. It may also help soothe earaches and provide relief from indigestion.

2. Cayenne Pepper

Cayenne pepper has anti-inflammatory properties, which are beneficial for the management of allergies, arthritis, and diabetes. It is also known to alleviate headaches, lower blood pressure, and promote healthy cholesterol levels. Additionally, cayenne pepper may encourage proper circulation in the body.

3. Cinnamon

Cinnamon boosts memory recall and is thought to improve cognition and has a regulatory effect on blood sugar, making it beneficial for those with type 2 diabetes. It is known for its cardiovascular benefits, as cinnamon consumption is thought to reduce the risk of heart attack and heart disease. It can also help to lower LDL cholesterol.

4. Clove

Clove has proven to be useful in the treatment of fungal infections such as ringworm. It is also a natural insect repellant when used in oil form. Cloves are also high in antioxidants, so it aids in protecting the body from illness and disease.

5. Dill

Dill has a calming effect and may be useful in the treatment of sleep problems such as insomnia. This herb is also known for its digestive aid; it promotes healthy digestion while also helping to treat digestion problems such as diarrhea or upset stomach.

6. Mint

Mint is known for its ability to relieve nausea, particularly when sipped in tea form. Mint also aids in digestion, providing relief from stomach cramps and discomfort associated with irritable bowel syndrome.

7. Oregano

Oregano is a natural source of omega-3, iron, potassium, and fiber. It is also an antibacterial that helps strengthen the body's immune system. It can also help shorten the duration and alleviate symptoms of a cold.

8. Rosemary

Rosemary is an herb that is high in antioxidants and also has anti-inflammatory, antifungal, and antiseptic properties, which makes it beneficial in treating and preventing a wide variety of health problems including skin infections and fungi. It also offers respiratory relief for those with chest colds or asthma.

9. Thyme

Thyme is rich in vitamins and minerals, which aid in promoting overall health. It is helpful, especially in oil or tea form, in treating congestion and coughs associated with croup, bronchitis, or other such illnesses. Thyme also promotes oral health when used as a rinse, and it helps improve bad breath.

10. Turmeric

Turmeric is a spice with antibacterial, anti-inflammatory, and antiseptic properties, which lends itself well to the treatment of minor cuts and scrapes. It may be beneficial in treating both skin conditions (such as psoriasis) and joint inflammation (such as arthritis).

Ten Super Ingredients

1. Apple Cider Vinegar

Apple cider vinegar can help cure heartburn, constipation, and indigestion. It can also help maintain healthy cholesterol and blood sugar levels. When diluted with water and applied topically, it serves as a natural acne and wart treatment.

2. Baking Soda

Baking soda has a soothing effect on skin when applied topically, as it helps relieve itching and redness. When diluted with water, it also settles an upset stomach. Additionally, it can help cure bad breath, as it rids the mouth of bacteria.

3. Cilantro

Cilantro is an herb that promotes healthy digestion and provides relief from gas and bloating. It settles the stomach and provides relief from nausea. Consumption of cilantro helps prevent urinary tract infections and also lowers bad cholesterol.

4. Coconut Oil

Applied topically, coconut oil moisturizes the skin and helps provide relief and healing from skin conditions like eczema and psoriasis and minor injuries like bumps and bruises. Coconut oil has antibacterial and antifungal properties, so it is beneficial in strengthening the immune system and building a resistance against new illnesses.

5. Ginger

Ginger is known for its ability to settle an upset stomach, providing relief from nausea and indigestion. Ginger is an antibacterial, antifungal, and antihistamine, so it is helpful in treating colds and allergies. It is an anti-inflammatory, so it may treat symptoms of arthritis.

6. Honey

Honey has antibacterial and antimicrobial properties, which makes it useful in the disinfection and healing of cuts, scrapes, and other minor skin injuries. Honey also provides relief from a cough and can help promote a restful night's sleep.

7. Mustard Seed

In addition to being a great source of omega-3, mustard seed is a natural anti-inflammatory, which is helpful in treating conditions such as asthma and arthritis. It helps promote a healthy gastrointestinal system and reduces the risk of associated types of cancer.

8. Olive Oil

Olive oil promotes heart and digestive health by lowering bad cholesterol and the risk of heart disease. When taken orally, it soothes a sore throat or cough and also helps treat and prevent constipation.

9. Sea Salt

Sea salt is beneficial in lowering high cholesterol and contrary to popular belief, high blood pressure. It may also treat asthma by decreasing inflammation of the respiratory system. Sea salt can also boost the immune system, thereby increasing the body's ability to fight off illnesses.

10. White Vinegar

Vinegar is thought to maintain and improve bone health, as it allows the body to absorb calcium more easily. It can also be used for cleansing the skin and treating existing conditions such as acne. Vinegar, taken orally in small doses, can also treat colds and coughs.

Ten Curative Foods and Beverages

1. Almond

Almonds are a food rich in vitamins and minerals and provide a host of cardiovascular benefits, including lowered cholesterol and reduced risk of heart disease. Almonds are also thought to improve cognitive development in children. Almonds may reduce the risk of obesity and diabetes.

2. Cranberry

Cranberries are beneficial in promoting a healthy urinary tract. They are also high in antioxidants, which help protect the body against illness and disease. Cranberries support kidney health and may prevent and treat kidney stones.

3. Elderberry

When taken in extract form, elderberry may help to shorten the duration and decrease the severity of the flu. Elderberry can boost the body's immune system and help the body respond quickly and strongly to viruses and infections. It is also known to relieve constipation.

4. Flaxseeds

Flaxseeds are rich in omega-3 and help prevent joint inflammation. They also help lower cholesterol and promote heart health. Flaxseeds are high in fiber and are therefore beneficial in treating and preventing constipation.

5. Garlic

Garlic is a natural antibiotic that helps treat bacterial and viral infections. It can also assist in maintaining healthy blood pressure and cholesterol levels. Consumption of garlic may also be linked to a lower risk of cancer.

6. Green Tea

Green tea is rich in antioxidants, which protect the body from illness and promote healthy cell growth. Drinking green tea is thought to boost immunity and lower the risk of many serious health conditions such as heart disease, arthritis, and certain cancers (like lung and breast cancer).

7. Lemon

Lemon is a fruit known to boost immunity with its antibacterial and antiviral properties. Lemons are rich in vitamin C and can help fight the common cold. Though its acidic nature may cause an initial burning sensation, lemon can help expedite the healing of a scratchy or sore throat.

8. Onion

The consumption of onions may help lower bad cholesterol. Onions also have antibacterial and antifungal properties and help break down mucus, making it beneficial for healing a sinus infection, cold, or other virus. Onion tea can promote a healthy respiratory system by relieving a cough and decreasing inflammation of the throat.

9. Salmon

Salmon is naturally high in omega-3 fatty acids, supporting neurological and cardiovascular health. Eating fish also promotes joint and tissue health through anti-inflammatory actions.

10. Yogurt

Yogurt supports digestive health and is known to help the body recover from conditions that affect digestion (such as diarrhea). It can also help lower bad cholesterol. Yogurt contains live cultures (probiotics) that promote the growth of healthy bacteria, which is particularly important when taking antibiotics that may kill both good and bad bacteria. Just be sure to pick from among the healthier yogurt brands without all the added sugars that can counteract the digestive benefits.

Ten Indispensable Oils

1. Chamomile

Chamomile oil has sedative properties that promote calmness and relaxation. When used in a bath or during massage, it can treat stress, headaches, and menstrual cramps. Chamomile oil, when diluted, also promotes a healthy scalp and may be useful in the treatment of lice.

2. Cinnamon

Cinnamon oil, when diluted, helps to promote circulation. It is also beneficial in topically treating infections, as it is an antibacterial and antiseptic agent. Cinnamon oil may also positively affect digestion and can treat diarrhea or an upset stomach.

3. Clove

Clove oil has disinfectant properties that make it particularly useful in treating minor cuts, scrapes, and burns. It is also proven to help relieve pain associated with a toothache. Diluted and applied topically, clove oil can be beneficial in the treatment of acne.

4. Eucalyptus

Eucalyptus oil is helpful in treating aches associated with a cold, flu, or minor muscle injuries. When eucalyptus oil is inhaled, it is thought to stimulate the senses in addition to helping to clear the nasal passages.

5. Fennel

Fennel oil is an expectorant that is also antibacterial, so it has the ability to treat and expedite the healing of a cough or cold. It provides relief from stomach problems such as nausea, bloating, or constipation. Fennel oil may also treat bacterial eye infections like conjunctivitis.

6. Lavender

Lavender oil is a useful form of aromatherapy, particularly in comforting children who have colic or who may be teething, as it promotes relaxation and sleep. Diluted lavender oil is also used to promote respiratory health in conditions that cause breathing problems, such as bronchitis, asthma, or sinusitis. Additionally, a massage with lavender oil will help soothe aching tissues and muscles.

7. Lemon

Lemon oil is thought to have a calming effect on the body; it stimulates the senses while also helping to relieve anxiety. Lemon oil is a natural insect repellant. When mixed with water, it can also be a beneficial skin treatment for eczema and acne.

8. Peppermint

Peppermint oil helps provide relief from headaches when used as a form of aromatherapy. Peppermint oil aromatherapy also helps clear nasal passages and promotes a healthy respiratory system. When diluted with water and sipped, it soothes an upset stomach associated with indigestion or gas.

9. Tea Tree

Tea tree oil is useful when applied topically to treat skin conditions such as acne or sunburn. It is also an antifungal that can be used to treat warts, ringworm, or athlete's foot. Tea tree oil can aid in recovery from congestion or other symptoms associated with viruses such as a cold or flu.

10. Ylang Ylang

Ylang ylang is an essential oil that may be beneficial in treating stress and anxiety, as it promotes relaxation and a sense of peace. When used as a form of aromatherapy, it may also help treat depression and restlessness.

Ten Vital Supplements

1. Calcium

Calcium is important in maintaining healthy bones and teeth, and it is especially important for young children with growing bodies. Proper calcium intake during youth can help prevent arthritis and osteoporosis in older age.

2. Coenzyme Q10

Coenzyme Q10 may be beneficial in the treatment of asthma, as it may have anti-inflammatory properties that promote bronchial health. It may also help treat symptoms of fatigue. Maintaining healthy levels of coenzyme Q10 may prove useful in preventing migraine headaches and promoting cardiovascular health.

3. Folate

Folate is beneficial in promoting healthy brain development. It is particularly important for fetal health to promote proper growth. Folate is also helpful in the treatment or prevention of both anemia and depression. Folic acid is a synthetic form of folate typically used in supplements and fortified foods.

4. Iron

Iron is crucial in assisting the transportation of oxygen throughout the body to the vital organs. Proper iron levels ward off anemia and fatigue while also promoting brain health. A healthy iron intake also helps treat and prevent insomnia and other sleep disorders.

5. Magnesium

Magnesium promotes neurological health; it can help treat and prevent headaches and migraines. It may also be useful in treating anxiety, stress, and depression. Magnesium provides support to the heart and may help lower the risk of high blood pressure, also known as hypertension. Magnesium is also effective in treating constipation.

6. Omega-3

Omega-3 fatty acids provide a host of benefits: anti-inflammation, lowered blood pressure, heart health, and improved heart and neurological functioning. Some studies suggest a link between omega-3s and relief of symptoms associated with bipolar disorder. Omega-3s are also thought to promote eye health and a lower risk of macular degeneration.

7. Vitamin B_{12}

Vitamin B_{12} is beneficial in preventing fatigue, anemia, and low energy. It also supports neurological health by decreasing symptoms associated with depression and anxiety. Vitamin B_{12} is also thought to lower the risk of stroke and certain cancers (such as lung or colon cancer).

8. Vitamin C

Vitamin C is a crucial antibacterial, antifungal, and antiviral vitamin that supports the immune system and reduces the severity and duration of an illness or infection. It helps to lower cholesterol and decreases the risk of cardiovascular and autoimmune diseases. Vitamin C also promotes healthy blood clotting.

9. Vitamin D

Vitamin D is important in maintaining proper bone health, as it is necessary in order for calcium to be properly absorbed. Vitamin D also supports a healthy immune system. It can aid in the treatment of serious conditions such as heart disease, diabetes, and kidney disease. Maintaining healthy vitamin D levels may prevent certain cancers and mental health disorders.

10. Zinc

Zinc is essential in boosting immunity and helps to reduce the severity and shorten the duration of both colds and cold sores. It is also beneficial in the treatment and healing of skin conditions such as psoriasis, acne, and eczema.

Ten Healing Herbs and Plants

1. Aloe

The gel from an aloe vera plant provides topical relief for skin problems such as minor burns or sunburns. It can also help to expedite healing cuts, blisters, and open sores. Aloe moisturizes the skin while also removing the sting associated with dermatological issues or injuries. Taken internally, aloe soothes the digestive tract.

2. Astragalus

Astragalus is a plant that helps boost the body's immune system, thereby providing an increased resistance to colds and viruses. It is also known to offer relief from heartburn and indigestion, as it regulates stomach acid.

3. Butterbur

The butterbur plant has natural anti-inflammatory properties that aid in the recovery of colds, sinus infections, and bronchial infections. It is also an expectorant that relieves a cough and makes breathing easier. Butterbur is also thought to be a natural treatment for recurring headaches including migraines.

4. Cacao

Cacao, the main ingredient in chocolate, comes from the Theobroma cacao tree and functions as a natural antioxidant. Antioxidants protect the body from illness and strengthen the immune system. Cacao is also thought to provide cardiovascular benefits and promotes healthy cholesterol levels.

5. Calendula

Calendula, from the marigold flower, is often used as an oil or ointment applied topically to relieve skin rashes and inflammation. It may also be used in tea form to reduce a fever and to soothe stomach ulcers.

6. Chamomile

Chamomile is a natural sedative that is beneficial when used to promote a sense of calm and relaxation, particularly at bedtime. It has also been shown to help treat the symptoms of irritable bowel syndrome by settling the stomach and promoting healthy bowel movements.

7. Echinacea

Echinacea is an herb that supports a healthy immune system. During an illness, it fights viruses and infections. When used topically, it also helps expedite the healing of minor injuries such as cuts, scrapes, and burns.

8. Eucalyptus

Eucalyptus leaves are helpful in expediting recovery from respiratory infections, as they provide relief from fever, cough, and congestion. Sipped as a tea, it can have a soothing effect on a sore throat.

9. Milk Thistle

Milk thistle is a plant that is primarily known to promote a healthy liver and detoxification, but it may also help to lower cholesterol. It may provide relief from pain associated with kidney stones as well.

10. Pelargonium

Pelargonium comes from the geranium plant and, when used in oil form, can treat dermatological conditions such as acne and eczema. It also has antibacterial and antifungal properties and has been shown to be quite effective in treating sinus and bronchial infections.

Ten Helpful Homeopathics

1. Antimonium Tartaricum

Antimonium tartaricum is a helpful homeopathic medicine that loosens thick mucus in children with a cough or chest cold. In doing so, coughs become more productive and the loosened mucus allows for easier breathing and swallowing.

2. Apis

Apis mellifica provides soothing relief following an insect sting or bite. It relieves the stinging sensation, redness, and swelling that may occur following such bites and stings. It is also useful for itchy skin conditions.

3. Arnica

Arnica montana provides first-aid relief for those experiencing pain associated with bumps and bruises. It also treats pulled or strained muscles and the aches and soreness that follow.

4. Belladonna

Belladonna is a plant with medicinal properties, though some parts of the plant are toxic. Belladonna relieves sinus pain that may occur with a sinus infection, cold, or allergies and is a common remedy for fevers.

5. Calcarea Phosphorica

Calcarea phosphorica in gel or tablet form helps alleviate pain and discomfort when a child is teething. It may also provide pain relief associated with normal childhood growing pains.

6. Carbo Vegetabilis

Carbo vegetabilis is a helpful ingredient in the treatment of babies experiencing colic. By reducing bloating, this homeopathic ingredient helps to relieve discomfort.

7. Euphrasia Officinalis

Euphrasia is a plant used to help treat eye infections or other eye conditions. It can be used to help treat redness, irritation, and swelling caused by allergies or conjunctivitis.

8. Pulsatilla

Pulsatilla is a type of flower that behaves as an expectorant and helps encourage recovery from a cold or sinus infection. It helps provide relief from a stuffy nose, earache, or sinus pressure.

9. Sulfur

Sulfur is a mineral that is helpful in treating skin conditions such as eczema or acne. It is used to help soothe red, itchy skin associated with these or other skin problems.

10. Thuja

Thuja is a type of tree that is useful in treating conditions that result from fungal infections. It is noted for its use in treating ringworm and warts when used topically. It may also be used to help infants and children cope with stressful medical procedures.

Ten Mind-Body Therapies

1. Acupuncture

Acupuncture is a key component of Traditional Chinese Medicine in which thin needles are inserted into specific parts of the body known as acupuncture points. Acupuncture is used to treat pain and to restore a natural balance in the body.

2. Biofeedback

Biofeedback is a noninvasive treatment option that is used to promote awareness of the state of one's physical or mental health. During biofeedback treatment, electrical sensors are applied to the body and various physiological parameters (e.g., heart rate, muscle tension, brain waves) are monitored. The feedback received from such monitoring helps provide the tools with which behavior and feelings may be modified, such as tics or anxieties.

3. Dance

Dance is a form of therapy that focuses on the relationship between the mind and body, combining physical movement and emotion. It can be used to help treat stress, anxiety, and sensory disorders.

4. Exercise

Regular exercise is extremely beneficial in children, as it allows them to expend their naturally high energy. It also serves as a physical outlet for anger, stress, and other emotions that may otherwise lead to behavioral problems. Outdoor free play may be particularly therapeutic.

5. Guided Imagery

Guided imagery is a technique that uses specific thought processes to manipulate a physical response. It can be helpful in trying to encourage a child to relax or fall asleep. This can be done by visualizing sensory details of a calm and peaceful scene, which often evokes a physical response from the body.

6. Hypnosis

Hypnosis is a form of therapy that combines concentration and relaxation in an effort to modify emotions or behavior. Hypnosis involves a trance-like state of consciousness, which can be useful in treating anxiety or depression. It may also help eliminate undesired behavior like bed-wetting.

7. Massage

Massage is a form of therapy that enables the body to relax while also working on the body's tissues. Massage is particularly helpful in treating soreness and discomfort associated with muscle or tissue injuries. It also promotes circulation and the relief of stress and tension.

8. Meditation

Meditation is a practice that involves intense focus in an effort to arrive at a place of self-awareness. It often homes in on breathing or concentrating on a specific focal point in order to achieve a goal, such as relief from pain or stress reduction. It may also help treat anxiety or depression.

9. Mindfulness-Based Stress Reduction (MBSR)

MBSR is a form of therapy that promotes an overall sense of awareness. It does not involve a single focal point or emotion but rather a mindfulness that covers all of the senses. It may be used to treat depression, stress, or anxiety as well as some neurological conditions that cause physical pain.

10. Yoga

Yoga uses stretching, specific physical positions, and breathing techniques to encourage relaxation, balance, and physical strength. Yoga is beneficial in the management of conditions such as ADHD/ADD, autism spectrum disorder, anxiety disorders, and mood disorders.

C

Treatment Alternatives A to Z

Welcome to the ultimate treatment alternative reference guide. This is a three-for-one special. First is an alphabetical listing by ailment. Second is an alphabetical listing by conventional remedy. Third is an alphabetical listing by natural and homeopathic treatment alternatives. So whether you've got in mind an ailment, a conventional remedy, or a treatment alternative, you can quickly find it and look up the associated information. Happy hunting!

Alphabetical by Ailment

Ailment	Conventional Remedy	Treatment Alternative
Acne	Proactiv Solutions	Poofy Organics Zippy Zit Zapper
ADHD/ADD	Ritalin	Neurofeedback
Allergies (seasonal)	Claritin	Ortho Molecular D-Hist Jr.
Anemia	Feosol	Floradix Iron + Herbs
Anger and tantrums	1-2-3 Magic	Free outdoor play
Anxiety/stress	Valium	Yoga
Asthma	Flovent MDI	Kan Herbals Deep Breath

Ailment	Conventional Remedy	Treatment Alternative
Athlete's foot	Desenex	New Chapter Garlic Force
Autism Spectrum Disorder	Risperdal	GFCF diet
Bad breath	Listerine	Klaire Ther-Biotic Complete Chewables
Bed-wetting	DDAVP	Hypnosis
Bee stings	Motrin	Boiron Apis Mellifica 30C
Bipolar disorder/mood regulation	Abilify	EMPower Plus
Bronchitis	Zithromax Children's Syrup	Umcka Cold Care
Bruises	Tylenol	Hyland's Bumps and Bruises
Burns	Silvadene	Aubrey Organic Pure Aloe Vera
Canker sores and cold sores	Blistex	Super Lysine+
Cavities	Luride	Spry Oral Rinse
Celiac disease and gluten intolerance	Gluten-Free Diet	VSL#3
Chicken pox	Benadryl	Aveeno Baby Soothing Bath Treatment
Colic	Mylicon	Traditional Medicinals Organic Chamomile Tea
Conjunctivitis (pinkeye)	Tobramycin	Boiron Optique 1
Constipation	Miralax	Bob's Red Mill Flaxseed Powder
Cough, dry	Robitussin	Boiron Chestal Cough Syrup

Ailment	Conventional Remedy	Treatment Alternative
Cough, wet	Dimetapp	Traditional Medicinals Organic Chamomile Tea
Coxsackie virus	Maalox/Benadryl/ Xylocaine (Viscous Lidocaine)	Traumeel-S
Cradle cap	Johnson's Baby Oil	Spectrum Organic Extra Virgin Olive Oil
Croup	Orapred	Young Living Eucalyptus Oil
Cuts and scrapes	Neosporin	Weleda Calendula Ointment
Dehydration	Gatorade Lemon-Lime Thirst Quencher	Zico Natural Bottled Pure Premium Coconut Water
Depression	Prozac	Nordic Naturals ProOmega Junior
Diaper rash	Balmex	California Baby Calendula Cream
Diarrhea	Imodium A-D	Florajen4Kids
Ear infection	Amoxil	HerbPharm Mullein Garlic
Earache	Children's Advil Suspension	Spectrum Organic Olive Oil
Eczema	Cortaid 1%	Atopiclair
Eye discharge	E-Mycin Ointment	Breastmilk
Failure to thrive	Pediasure	Pediasmart
Fatigue	BOOST	Prothera MitoThera
Fever	Tylenol	Water
Flu	Tamiflu	Sambucol
Food allergies	Benadryl	Klaire Ther-Biotic Infant

Ailment	Conventional Remedy	Treatment Alternative
GERD/reflux/ heartburn	Nexium	Lee Silsby Enhansa
Growing pains	Tylenol	Carlson for Kids D Drops
Head lice	Nix	LiceMD
High cholesterol	Lipitor	Nordic Naturals ProOmega
Hives	Benadryl	Traditional Medicinals Organic Nettle Leaf Tea
Impetigo	Bactroban	HNZ Bio Active Manuka Honey
Insect bites	Lanacane Anti-itch	Arm and Hammer Baking Soda
Irritable bowel syndrome	Bentyl	Nature's Way Pepogest
Joint pains	Advil	Pure Encapsulations Boswellia AKBA
Kidney stones	Lithotripsy	Lemon juice
Labial adhesions	Premarin Cream	Weleda Calendula Ointment
Menstrual cramps	Anaprox	BlueBonnet Vitamin B1
Migraine headache	Topamax	Petadolex
Minor skin infections	Bactine	Jason 45000IU Vitamin E Pure Beauty Oil
Molluscum	Liquid nitrogen	Tea Tree Therapy Lemon Myrtle 100% Essential Oil
Mononucleosis	Deltasone	Carlson for Kids Chewable Vitamin C
Motion sickness	Dramamine	New Chapter Ginger Force
Muscle aches	Aleve	Boiron Arnica Gel

Ailment	Conventional Remedy	Treatment Alternative
Nausea/vomiting	Zofran	Sea Bands
Night terrors	Observation	Floradix Iron + Herbs
Nosebleeds	Neo-Synephrine	NeilMed NasoGel
Obsessive- compulsive disorder	Zoloft	Cognitive behavioral therapy
Pneumonia	Ceftin	Thorne Research Zinc Sulfate
Poison ivy	Orapred	All Terrain Poison Ivy/Oak Cream
Psoriasis	Valisone	Dovonex Ointment
Recurrent abdominal pain	Elavil	Hypnotherapy
Ringworm	Diflucan	Aroma MD Tea Tree Oil
Runny nose	Triaminic Cold & Allergy Syrup	Boiron Coldcalm
Seizures	Trileptal	Neurofeedback
Sinusitis (sinus infection)	Augmentin	HerbPharm Andrographis Extract
Sleep problems	Catapres	Pure Encapsulations Melatonin
Sore throat	Cepacol	Traditional Medicinals Organic Throat Coat Tea
Speech development/ stuttering	Speech Therapy	SPEAK Capsules
Spitting up	Zantac	Dairy elimination
Sprains	Aleve	Burt's Bees Res-Q Ointment
Stuffy nose	Sudafed	Little Noses Saline Spray

Ailment	Conventional Remedy	Treatment Alternative
Sunburn	Solarcaine Spray	Jason Aloe Vera 84% Moisturizing Cream
Swimmer's ear	Ciprodex	Spectrum Naturals Organic Apple Cider Vinegar
Swollen glands (nodes)	Augmentin	Lymph massage
Teething	Baby Orajel	Boiron Camilia
Tension headache	Motrin	Acupuncture
Thrush	Bio-Statin	Klaire Infant Ther-Biotic Complete
Tics/Tourette's syndrome	Tenex	Hypnosis
Umbilical cord care	Rubbing alcohol	Air
Urinary tract infection	Septra	HerbPharm Cranberry Extract
Warts	Compound W	Tyco Duct Tape

Alphabetical by Conventional Remedy

Conventional Remedy	Treatment Alternative	Ailment
1-2-3 Magic	Free outdoor play	Anger and tantrums
Abilify	EMPower Plus	Bipolar disorder/mood regulation
Advil	Pure Encapsulations Boswellia AKBA	Joint pains
Aleve	Boiron Arnica Gel	Muscle aches
Aleve	Burt's Bees Res-Q Ointment	Sprains

Conventional Remedy	Treatment Alternative	Ailment
Amoxil	HerbPharm Mullein Garlic	Ear infection
Anaprox	BlueBonnet Vitamin B_1	Menstrual cramps
Augmentin	HerbPharm Andrographis Extract	Sinusitis (sinus infection)
Augmentin	Lymph massage	Swollen glands (nodes)
Advil (Children's Suspension)	Spectrum Organic Olive Oil	Earache
Bactine	Jason 45000IU Vitamin E Pure Beauty Oil	Minor skin infections
Bactroban	HNZ Bio Active Manuka Honey	Impetigo
Balmex	California Baby Calendula Cream	Diaper rash
Benadryl	Aveeno Baby Soothing Bath Treatment	Chicken pox
Benadryl	Klaire Ther-Biotic Infant	Food allergies
Benadryl	Traditional Medicinals Organic Nettle Leaf Tea	Hives
Bentyl	Nature's Way Pepogest	Irritable bowel syndrome
Bio-Statin	Klaire Infant Ther-Biotic Complete	Thrush
Blistex	Super Lysine+	Canker sores and cold sores
BOOST	Prothera MitoThera	Fatigue
Catapres	Pure Encapsulations Melatonin	Sleep problems

Conventional Remedy	Treatment Alternative	Ailment
Ceftin	Thorne Research Zinc Sulfate	Pneumonia
Cepacol	Traditional Medicinals Organic Throat Coat Tea	Sore throat
Ciprodex	Spectrum Naturals Organic Apple Cide Vinegar	Swimmer's ear
Claritin	Ortho Molecular D-Hist Jr.	Allergies (seasonal)
Compound W	Tyco Duct Tape	Warts
Cortaid 1%	Atopiclair	Eczema
DDAVP	Hypnosis	Bed-wetting
Deltasone	Carlson for Kids Chewable Vitamin C	Mononucleosis
Desenex	New Chapter Garlic Force	Athlete's foot
Diflucan	Aroma MD Tea Tree Oil	Ringworm
Dimetapp	Traditional Medicinals Organic Chamomile Tea	Cough, wet
Dramamine	New Chapter Ginger Force	Motion sickness
E-Mycin Ointment	Breastmilk	Eye discharge
Elavil	Hypnotherapy	Recurrent abdominal pain
Feosol	Floradix Iron + Herbs	Anemia
Flovent MDI	Kan Herbals Deep Breath	Asthma
Gatorade	Zico Natural Bottled Pure Premium CW	Dehydration
Gluten-free diet	VSL#3	Celiac disease/gluten intolerance
Imodium A-D	Florajen4Kids	Diarrhea

Conventional Remedy	Treatment Alternative	Ailment
Johnson's Baby Oil	Spectrum Organic Extra Virgin Olive Oil	Cradle cap
Lanacane Anti-Itch	Arm and Hammer Baking Soda	Insect bites
Lipitor	Nordic Naturals ProOmega	High cholesterol
Liquid nitrogen	Tea Tree Therapy Lemon Myrtle 100% Essential Oil	Molluscum
Listerine	Klaire Ther-Biotic Complete Chewables	Bad breath
Lithotripsy	Lemon juice	Kidney stones
Luride	Spry Oral Rinse	Cavities
Maalox/Benadryl/(Viscous Lidocaine)	Traumeel-S	Coxsackie virus
Miralax	Bob's Red Mill Flaxseed Powder	Constipation
Motrin	Acupuncture	Tension headache
Motrin	Boiron Apis Mellifica 30C	Bee stings
Mylicon	Traditional Medicinals Organic Chamomile Tea	Colic
Neo-Synephrine	NeilMed NasoGel	Nosebleeds
Neosporin	Weleda Calendula Ointment	Cuts and scrapes
Nexium	Lee Silsby Enhansa	GERD/reflux/heartburn
Nix	LiceMD	Head lice
Observation	Floradix Iron + Herbs	Night terrors
Orajel (Baby)	Boiron Camilia	Teething

Conventional Remedy	Treatment Alternative	Ailment
Orapred	All Terrain Poison Ivy/Oak Cream	Poison ivy
Pediasure	Pediasmart	Failure to thrive
Prelone	Young Living Eucalyptus Oil	Croup
Premarin Cream	Weleda Calendula Ointment	Labial adhesions
Proactiv	Poofy Organics	Acne Zippy Zit Zapper
Prozac	Nordic Naturals Ultimate Omega Junior	Depression
Risperdal	GFCF diet	Autism Spectrum Disorder
Ritalin	Neurofeedback	ADHD/ADD
Robitussin	Boiron Chestal	Cough, dry
Rubbing alcohol	Air	Umbilical cord care
Silvadene	Aubrey Organic Pure Aloe Vera	Burns
Solarcaine Spray	Jason Aloe Vera 84% Moisturizing Cream	Sunburn
Speech therapy	SPEAK Capsules	Speech development/ stuttering
Sudafed	NeilMed NasoFlo Neti Pot	Stuffy nose
Septra	HerbPharm Cranberry Extract	Urinary tract infection
Tamiflu	Sambucol	Flu
Tenex	Hypnosis	Tics/Tourette's syndrome
Tobramycin	Boiron Optique 1	Conjunctivitis (pinkeye)

Conventional Remedy	Treatment Alternative	Ailment
Topamax	Petadolex	Migraine headache
Triaminic Cold & Allergy Syrup	Boiron Coldcalm	Runny nose
Trileptal	Neurofeedback	Seizures
Tylenol	Carlson for Kids D Drops	Growing pains
Tylenol	Hyland's Bumps and Bruises	Bruises
Tylenol	Water	Fever
Valisone	Dovonex Ointment	Psoriasis
Valium	Yoga	Anxiety/stress
Zantac	Dairy elimination	Spitting up
Zithromax	Umcka Cold Care Children's Syrup	Bronchitis
Zofran	Sea Bands	Nausea/vomiting
Zoloft	Cognitive behavioral therapy	Obsessive-compulsive disorder

Alphabetical by Treatment Alternative

Treatment Alternative	Conventional Remedy	Ailment
Acupuncture	Motrin	Tension headache
Air	Rubbing alcohol	Umbilical cord care
All Terrain Poison Ivy/Oak Cream	Orapred	Poison ivy
Arm and Hammer Baking Soda	Lanacane Anti-Itch	Insect bites
Aroma MD Tea Tree Oil	Diflucan	Ringworm
Atopiclair	Cortaid 1%	Eczema
Aubrey Organic Pure Aloe Vera	Silvadene	Burns
Aveeno Baby Soothing Bath Treatment	Benadryl	Chicken pox
BlueBonnet Vitamin B1	Anaprox	Menstrual cramps
Bob's Red Mill Flaxseed Powder	Miralax	Constipation
Boiron Apis Mellifica 30C	Motrin	Bee stings
Boiron Arnica Gel	Aleve	Muscle aches
Boiron Camilia	Tylenol	Teething
Boiron Chestal	Robitussin	Cough, dry
Boiron Chestal Cough Syrup	Dimetapp	Cough, wet
Boiron Coldcalm	Triaminic Cold & Allergy Syrup	Runny nose
Boiron Optique 1	Tobramycin	Conjunctivitis (pinkeye)
Breastmilk	E-Mycin Ointment	Eye discharge

Treatment Alternative	Conventional Remedy	Ailment
Burt's Bees Res-Q Ointment	Aleve	Sprains
California Baby Calendula Cream	Balmex	Diaper rash
Carlson for Kids Chewable Vitamin C	Deltasone	Mononucleosis
Carlson for Kids D Drops	Tylenol	Growing pains
Cognitive behavioral therapy	Zoloft	Obsessive-compulsive disorder
Dairy elimination	Zantac	Spitting up
Dovonex Ointment	Valisone	Psoriasis
EMPower Plus	Abilify	Bipolar disorder/mood regulation
Floradix Iron + Herbs	Feosol	Anemia
Floradix Iron+ Herbs	Observation	Night terrors
Florajen4Kids	Imodium A-D	Diarrhea
Free outdoor play	1-2-3 Magic	Anger and tantrums
GFCF diet	Risperdal	Autism Spectrum Disorder
HerbPharm Andrographis Extract	Augmentin	Sinusitis (sinus infection)
HerbPharm Cranberry Extract	Suprax	Urinary tract infection
HerbPharm Mullein Garlic	Amoxil	Ear infection
HNZ Bio Active Manuka Honey	Bactroban	Impetigo
Hyland's Bumps and Bruises	Tylenol	Bruises

Treatment Alternative	Conventional Remedy	Ailment
Hypnosis	DDAVP	Bed-wetting
Hypnosis	Tenex	Tics/Tourette's syndrome
Hypnotherapy	Elavil	Recurrent abdominal pain
Jason 45000IU Vitamin E Pure Beauty Oil	Bactine	Minor skin infections
Jason Aloe Vera 84% Moisturizing Cream	Solarcaine Spray	Sunburn
Kan Herbals Deep Breath	Flovent MDI	Asthma
Klaire Infant Ther-Biotic Complete	Bio-Statin	Thrush
Klaire Ther-Biotic Complete Chewables	Listerine	Bad breath
Klaire Ther-Biotic Infant	Benadryl	Food allergies
Lee Silsby Enhansa	Nexium	GERD/reflux/Heartburn
Lemon juice	Lithotripsy	Kidney stones
LiceMD	Nix	Head lice
Little Noses Saline Spray	Sudafed	Stuffy nose
Lymph massage	Augmentin	Swollen glands (nodes)
Nature's Way Pepogest	Bentyl	Irritable bowel syndrome
NeilMed NasoGel	Neo-Synephrine	Nosebleeds
Neurofeedback	Ritalin	ADHD/ADD
Neurofeedback	Trileptal	Seizures
New Chapter Garlic Force	Desenex	Athlete's foot
New Chapter Ginger Force	Dramamine	Motion sickness
Nordic Naturals ProOmega	Lipitor	High cholesterol

Treatment Alternative	Conventional Remedy	Ailment
Nordic Naturals ProOmega Junior	Prozac	Depression
Ortho Molecular D-Hist Jr.	Claritin	Allergies (seasonal)
Pediasmart	Pediasure	Failure to thrive
Petadolex	Topamax	Migraine headache
Poofy Organics Zippy Zit Zapper	Proactiv	Acne
Prothera MitoThera	Sugar, caffeine	Fatigue
Pure Encapsulations Boswellia AKBA	Advil	Joint pains
Pure Encapsulations Melatonin	Catapres	Sleep problems
Sambucol	Tamiflu	Flu
Sea Bands	Zofran	Nausea/vomiting
SPEAK Capsules	Speech therapy	Speech development/ stuttering
Spectrum Naturals Organic Apple Cider Vinegar	Ciprodex	Swimmer's ear
Spectrum Organic Olive Oil	Advil (Children's Suspension)	Earache
Spectrum Organic Extra Virgin Olive Oil	Johnson's Baby Oil	Cradle cap
Spry Oral Rinse	Luride	Cavities
Super Lysine+	Blistex	Canker sores and cold sores
Tea Tree Therapy Lemon Myrtle 100% Essential Oil	Liquid nitrogen	Molluscum

Treatment Alternative	Conventional Remedy	Ailment
Thorne Research Zinc Sulfate	Ceftin	Pneumonia
Traditional Medicinals Organic Chamomile Tea	Mylicon	Colic
Traditional Medicinals Organic Nettle Leaf Tea	Benadryl	Hives
Traditional Medicinals Organic Throat Coat Tea	Tylenol	Sore throat
Traumeel-S	Maalox/Benadryl/ Xylocaine (Viscous Lidocaine)	Coxsackie virus
Tyco Duct Tape	Compound W	Warts
Umcka Cold Care Children's Syrup	Zithromax	Bronchitis
VSL#3	Gluten-free Diet	Celiac disease/gluten intolerance
Water	Tylenol	Fever
Weleda Calendula Ointment	Neosporin	Cuts and scrapes
Weleda Calendula Ointment	Premarin Cream	Labial adhesions
Yoga	Valium	Anxiety/stress
Young Living Eucalyptus Oil	Orapred	Croup
Zico Natural Bottled Pure Premium Coconut Water	Gatorade Lemon-Lime	Dehydration

D

Citations for *Science Says* Sidebars

Chapter 1: Baby Matters

Colic

Savino F, Cresi F, Castagno E, Silvestro L, Oggero R. A randomized double-blind placebo-controlled trial of a standardized extract of Matricaria recutita, Foeniculum vulgare, and Melissa officinalis (ColiMil) in the treatment of breastfed colicky infants. Phytother Res. 2005 Apr;19(4):335-40.

Cradle Cap

Geweely N. Antifungal Activity of Ozonized Olive Oil (Oleozone). Int. J. Agri. Biol., Vol. 8, No. 5, 2006, available at http://www.fspublishers.org/ijab/past-issues/IJABVOL_8_NO_5/24.pdf, accessed March 23, 2012.

Diaper Rash

Preethi KC, Kuttan R. Wound healing activity of flower extract of Calendula officinalis. J Basic Clin Physiol Pharmacol. 2009;20(1):73-9.

Eye Discharge (Blocked Tear Ducts)

Verd S. Switch from antibiotic eye drops to instillation of mother's milk drops as a treatment of infant epiphora. J Trop Pediatr. 2007 Feb;53(1):68-9.

Spitting Up (Baby Reflux)

Cavataio F, Carroccio A, Iacono G. Milk-induced reflux in infants less than one year of age. J Pediatr Gastroenterol Nutr. 2000;30 Suppl:S36-44.

Teething

Bhaskaran N, Shukla S, Srivastava JK, Gupta S. Chamomile: an anti-inflammatory agent inhibits inducible nitric oxide synthase expression by blocking RelA/p65 activity. Int J Mol Med. 2010 Dec;26(6):935-40.

Thrush

Hasslöf P, Hedberg M, Twetman S, Stecksén-Blicks C. Growth inhibition of oral mutans streptococci and candida by commercial probiotic lactobacilli—an in vitro study. BMC Oral Health. 2010 Jul 2;10:18.

Umbilical Cord Care

Dore S, Buchan D, Coulas S, Hamber L, Stewart M, Cowan D, Jamieson L. Alcohol versus natural drying for newborn cord care. J Obstet Gynecol Neonatal Nurs. 1998 Nov-Dec;27(6):621-7.

Chapter 2: Watch Your Mouth

Bad Breath

Iwamoto T, Suzuki N, Tanabe K, Takeshita T, Hirofuji T. Effects of probiotic Lactobacillus salivarius WB21 on halitosis and oral health: an open-label pilot trial. Oral Surg Oral Med Oral Pathol Oral Radiol Endod. 2010 Aug;110(2):201-8.

Canker Sores and Cold Sores

Singh BB, Udani J, Vinjamury SP, Der-Martirosian C, Gandhi S, Khorsan R, Nanjegowda D, Singh V. Safety and effectiveness of an L-lysine, zinc, and herbal-based product on the treatment of facial and circumoral herpes. Altern Med Rev. 2005 Jun;10(2):123-7.

Cavities

Milgrom P, Ly KA, Tut OK, Mancl L, Roberts MC, Briand K, Gancio MJ. Xylitol pediatric topical oral syrup to prevent dental caries: a double-blind randomized clinical trial of efficacy. Arch Pediatr Adolesc Med. 2009 Jul;163(7):601-7.

Coxsackie Virus

Oberbaum M, Yaniv I, Ben-Gal Y, Stein J, Ben-Zvi N, Freedman LS, Branski D. A randomized, controlled clinical trial of the homeopathic medication TRAUMEEL S in the treatment of chemotherapy-induced stomatitis in children undergoing stem cell transplantation. Cancer. 2001 Aug 1;92(3):684-90.

Sore Throat

Brinckmann J, Sigwart H, van Houten Taylor L. Safety and efficacy of a traditional herbal medicine (Throat Coat) in symptomatic temporary relief of pain in patients with acute pharyngitis: a multicenter, prospective, randomized, double-blinded, placebo-controlled study. J Altern Complement Med. 2003 Apr;9(2):285-98.

Swollen Glands (Nodes)

Bernas M, Witte M, Kriederman B, Summers P, Witte C. Massage therapy in the treatment of lymphedema. Rationale, results, and applications. IEEE Eng Med Biol Mag. 2005 Mar-Apr;24(2):58-68.

Chapter 3: Seeing, Hearing, and Smelling

Conjunctivitis (Pinkeye)

Stoss M, Michels C, Peter E, Beutke R, Gorter RW. Prospective cohort trial of Euphrasia single-dose eye drops in conjunctivitis. J Altern Complement Med. 2000 Dec;6(6):499-508.

Earache

Lucas L, Russell A, Keast R. Molecular mechanisms of inflammation. Anti-inflammatory benefits of virgin olive oil and the phenolic compound oleocanthal. Curr Pharm Des. 2011;17(8):754-68.

Ear Infection

Sarrell EM, Cohen HA, Kahan E. Naturopathic treatment for ear pain in children. Pediatrics. 2003 May;111(5 Pt 1):e574-9.

Runny Nose

Ramchandani NM. Homeopathic treatment of upper respiratory tract infections in children: evaluation of thirty case series. Complement Ther Clin Pract. 2010 May;16(2):101-8.

Sinusitis (Sinus Infection)

Gabrielian ES, Shukarian AK, Goukasova GI, Chandanian GL, Panossian AG, Wikman G, Wagner H. A double blind, placebo-controlled study of Andrographis paniculata fixed combination Kan Jang in the treatment of acute upper respiratory tract infections including sinusitis. Phytomedicine. 2002 Oct;9(7):589-97.

Stuffy Nose

Wang YH, Yang CP, Ku MS, Sun HL, Lue KH. Efficacy of nasal irrigation in the treatment of acute sinusitis in children. Int J Pediatr Otorhinolaryngol. 2009 Dec;73(12):1696-701.

Swimmer's Ear

Kaushik V, Malik T, Saeed SR. Interventions for acute otitis externa. Cochrane Database Syst Rev. 2010 Jan 20;(1):CD004740.

Chapter 4: Take Your Breath Away

Allergies (Seasonal)

1. Park HH, Lee S, Son HY, Park SB, Kim MS, Choi EJ, Singh TS, Ha JH, Lee MG, Kim JE, Hyun MC, Kwon TK, Kim YH, Kim SH. Flavonoids inhibit histamine release and expression of proinflammatory cytokines in mast cells. Arch Pharm Res. 2008 Oct;31(10):1303-11.

2. Roschek B Jr, Fink RC, McMichael M, Alberte RS. Nettle extract (Urtica dioica) affects key receptors and enzymes associated with allergic rhinitis. Phytother Res. 2009 Jul;23(7):920-6.

3. N-acetylcysteine. Altern Med Rev. 2000 Oct;5(5):467-71.

Asthma

Li XM, Brown L. Efficacy and mechanisms of action of traditional Chinese medicines for treating asthma and allergy. J Allergy Clin Immunol. 2009 Feb;123(2):297-306; quiz 307-8.

Bronchitis

Matthys H, Kamin W, Funk P, Heger M. Pelargonium sidoides preparation (EPs 7630) in the treatment of acute bronchitis in adults and children. Phytomedicine. 2007;14 Suppl 6:69-73.

Dry Cough

1. Haidvogl M, Riley DS, Heger M, Brien S, Jong M, Fischer M, Lewith GT, Jansen G, Thurneysen AE. Homeopathic and conventional treatment for acute respiratory and ear complaints: a comparative study on outcome in the primary care setting. BMC Complement Altern Med. 2007 Mar 2;7:7.

2. Shadkam MN, Mozaffari-Khosravi H, Mozayan MR. A comparison of the effect of honey, dextromethorphan, and diphenhydramine on nightly cough and sleep quality in children and their parents. J Altern Complement Med. 2010 Jul;16(7):787-93.

Wet Cough

Haggag EG, Abou-Moustafa MA, Boucher W, Theoharides TC. The effect of a herbal water-extract on histamine release from mast cells and on allergic asthma. J Herb Pharmacother. 2003;3(4):41-54.

Croup

Ben-Arye E, Dudai N, Eini A, Torem M, Schiff E, Rakover Y. Treatment of upper respiratory tract infections in primary care: a randomized study using aromatic herbs. Evid Based Complement Alternat Med. 2011;2011:690346.

Pneumonia

Valavi E, Hakimzadeh M, Shamsizadeh A, Aminzadeh M, Alghasi A. The efficacy of zinc supplementation on outcome of children with severe pneumonia. A randomized double-blind placebo-controlled clinical trial. Indian J Pediatr. 2011 Sep;78(9):1079-84.

Chapter 5: Temperature Rising

Fever

Section on Clinical Pharmacology and Therapeutics; Committee on Drugs, Sullivan JE, Farrar HC. Fever and antipyretic use in children. Pediatrics. 2011 Mar;127(3):580-7.

Flu

Zakay-Rones Z, Thom E, Wollan T, Wadstein J. Randomized study of the efficacy and safety of oral elderberry extract in the treatment of influenza A and B virus infections. J Int Med Res. 2004 Mar-Apr;32(2):132-40.

Mononucleosis

Uesato S, Kitagawa Y, Kaijima T, Tokuda H, Okuda M, Mou XY, Mukainaka T, Nishino H. Inhibitory effects of 6-O-acylated L-ascorbic acids possessing a straight- or branched-acyl chain on Epstein-Barr virus activation. Cancer Lett. 2001 May 26;166(2):143-6.

Chapter 6: Tummy Troubles

Constipation

Tabbers MM, Boluyt N, Berger MY, Benninga MA. Nonpharmacologic treatments for childhood constipation: systematic review. Pediatrics. 2011 Oct;128(4):753-61.

Diarrhea

Allen SJ, Martinez EG, Gregorio GV, Dans LF. Probiotics for treating acute infectious diarrhoea. Cochrane Database Syst Rev. 2010 Nov 10;(11):CD003048.

GERD/Reflux/Heartburn

Rafiee P, Nelson VM, Manley S, Wellner M, Floer M, Binion DG, Shaker R. Effect of curcumin on acidic pH-induced expression of IL-6 and IL-8 in human esophageal epithelial cells (HET-1A): role of PKC, MAPKs, and NF-kappaB. Am J Physiol Gastrointest Liver Physiol. 2009 Feb;296(2):G388-98.

Irritable Bowel Syndrome

Kline RM, Kline JJ, Di Palma J, Barbero GJ. Enteric-coated, pH-dependent peppermint oil capsules for the treatment of irritable bowel syndrome in children. J Pediatr. 2001 Jan;138(1):125-8.

Motion Sickness

Lien HC, Sun WM, Chen YH, Kim H, Hasler W, Owyang C. Effects of ginger on motion sickness and gastric slow-wave dysrhythmias induced by circular vection. Am J Physiol Gastrointest Liver Physiol. 2003 Mar;284(3):G481-9.

Nausea/Vomiting

Lee A, Fan LT. Stimulation of the wrist acupuncture point P6 for preventing postoperative nausea and vomiting. Cochrane Database Syst Rev. 2009 Apr 15;(2):CD003281.

Recurrent Abdominal Pain

Vlieger AM, Menko-Frankenhuis C, Wolfkamp SC, Tromp E, Benninga MA. Hypnotherapy for children with functional abdominal pain or irritable bowel syndrome: a randomized controlled trial. Gastroenterology. 2007 Nov;133(5):1430-6.

Chapter 7: Eating and Energy

Anemia

Shamah-Levy T, Villalpando S, Rivera-Dommarco JA, Mundo-Rosas V, Cuevas-Nasu L, Jiménez-Aguilar A. Ferrous gluconate and ferrous sulfate added to a complementary food distributed by the Mexican nutrition program Oportunidades have a comparable efficacy to reduce iron deficiency in toddlers. J Pediatr Gastroenterol Nutr. 2008 Nov;47(5):660-6.

Celiac Disease/Gluten Intolerance

1. De Angelis M, Rizzello CG, Fasano A, Clemente MG, De Simone C, Silano M, De Vincenzi M, Losito I, Gobbetti M. VSL#3 probiotic preparation has the capacity to hydrolyze gliadin polypeptides responsible for Celiac Sprue. Biochim Biophys Acta. 2006 Jan;1762(1):80-93.

2. Domínguez-Muñoz JE. Pancreatic enzyme replacement therapy for pancreatic exocrine insufficiency: when is it indicated, what is the goal and how to do it? Adv Med Sci. 2011;56(1):1-5.

Failure to Thrive

Bray GA, Nielsen SJ, Popkin BM. Consumption of high-fructose corn syrup in beverages may play a role in the epidemic of obesity. Am J Clin Nutr. 2004 Apr;79(4):537-43.

Fatigue

Sun M, Qian F, Shen W, Tian C, Hao J, Sun L, Liu J. Mitochondrial nutrients stimulate performance and mitochondrial biogenesis in exhaustively exercised rats. Scand J Med Sci Sports. 2011 Apr 21.

Davis JM, Carlstedt CJ, Chen S, Carmichael MD, Murphy EA. The dietary flavonoid quercetin increases VO(2max) and endurance capacity. Int J Sport Nutr Exerc Metab. 2010 Feb;20(1):56-62.

Food Allergies

Kukkonen K, Kuitunen M, Haahtela T, Korpela R, Poussa T, Savilahti E. High intestinal IgA associates with reduced risk of IgE-associated allergic diseases. Pediatr Allergy Immunol. 2010 Feb;21(1 Pt 1):67-73.

High Cholesterol

O'Sullivan TA, Ambrosini GL, Mori TA, Beilin LJ, Oddy WH. Omega-3 Index correlates with healthier food consumption in adolescents and with reduced cardiovascular disease risk factors in adolescent boys. Lipids. 2011 Jan;46(1):59-67.

Chapter 8: Midsection Maladies

Bed-wetting

Edwards SD, van der Spuy HI. Hypnotherapy as a treatment for enuresis. J Child Psychol Psychiatry. 1985 Jan;26(1):161-70.

Banerjee S, Srivastav A, Palan BM. Hypnosis and self-hypnosis in the management of nocturnal enuresis: a comparative study with imipramine therapy. Am J Clin Hypn. 1993 Oct;36(2):113-9.

Kidney Stones

Cicerello E, Merlo F, Maccatrozzo L. Urinary alkalization for the treatment of uric acid nephrolithiasis. Arch Ital Urol Androl. 2010 Sep;82(3):145-8.

Labial Adhesions

Preethi KC, Kuttan G, Kuttan R. Anti-inflammatory activity of flower extract of Calendula officinalis Linn. and its possible mechanism of action. Indian J Exp Biol. 2009 Feb;47(2):113-20.

Della Loggia R, Tubaro A, Sosa S, Becker H, Saar S, Isaac O. The role of triterpenoids in the topical anti-inflammatory activity of Calendula officinalis flowers. Planta Med. 1994 Dec;60(6):516-20.

Menstrual Cramps

Proctor ML, Murphy PA. Herbal and dietary therapies for primary and secondary dysmenorrhoea. Cochrane Database Syst Rev. 2001;(3):CD002124.

Urinary Tract Infections

Ferrara P, Romaniello L, Vitelli O, Gatto A, Serva M, Cataldi L. Cranberry juice for the prevention of recurrent urinary tract infections: a randomized controlled trial in children. Scand J Urol Nephrol. 2009;43(5):369-72.

Di Martino P, Agniel R, David K, Templer C, Gaillard JL, Denys P, Botto H. Reduction of Escherichia coli adherence to uroepithelial bladder cells after consumption of cranberry juice: a double-blind randomized placebo-controlled cross-over trial. World J Urol. 2006 Feb;24(1):21-7.

Chapter 9: Dermatological Dilemmas

Acne

Enshaieh S, Jooya A, Siadat AH, Iraji F. The efficacy of 5% topical tea tree oil gel in mild to moderate acne vulgaris: a randomized, double-blind placebo-controlled study. Indian J Dermatol Venereol Leprol. 2007 Jan-Feb;73(1):22-5.

Athlete's Foot

Ledezma E, DeSousa L, Jorquera A, Sanchez J, Lander A, Rodriguez E, Jain MK, Apitz-Castro R. Efficacy of ajoene, an organosulphur derived from garlic, in the short-term therapy of tinea pedis. Mycoses. 1996 Sep-Oct;39(9-10):393-5.

Chicken Pox

Kurtz ES, Wallo W. Colloidal oatmeal: history, chemistry and clinical properties. J Drugs Dermatol. 2007 Feb;6(2):167-70.

Eczema

Saeedi M, Morteza-Semnani K, Ghoreishi MR. The treatment of atopic dermatitis with licorice gel. J Dermatolog Treat. 2003 Sep;14(3):153-7.

Head Lice

Heukelbach J, Pilger D, Oliveira FA, Khakban A, Ariza L, Feldmeier H. A highly efficacious pediculicide based on dimeticone: randomized observer blinded comparative trial. BMC Infect Dis. 2008 Sep 10;8:115.

Impetigo

Willix DJ, Molan PC, Harfoot CG. A comparison of the sensitivity of wound-infecting species of bacteria to the antibacterial activity of manuka honey and other honey. J Appl Bacteriol. 1992 Nov;73(5):388-94.

Minor Skin Infections

Zampieri N, Zuin V, Burro R, Ottolenghi A, Camoglio FS. A prospective study in children: Pre- and post-surgery use of vitamin E in surgical incisions. J Plast Reconstr Aesthet Surg. 2010 Sep;63(9):1474-8.

Molluscum

Burke BE, Baillie JE, Olson RD. Essential oil of Australian lemon myrtle (Backhousia citriodora) in the treatment of molluscum contagiosum in children. Biomed Pharmacother. 2004 May;58(4):245-7.

Psoriasis

de Jager ME, de Jong EM, van de Kerkhof PC, Seyger MM. Efficacy and safety of treatments for childhood psoriasis: a systematic literature review. J Am Acad Dermatol. 2010 Jun;62(6):1013-30.

Ringworm

Barchiesi F, Silvestri C, Arzeni D, Ganzetti G, Castelletti S, Simonetti O, Cirioni O, Kamysz W, Kamysz E, Spreghini E, Abruzzetti A, Riva A, Offidani AM, Giacometti A, Scalise G. In vitro susceptibility of dermatophytes to conventional and alternative antifungal agents. Med Mycol. 2009 May;47(3):321-6.

Warts

Focht DR 3rd, Spicer C, Fairchok MP. The efficacy of duct tape vs cryotherapy in the treatment of verruca vulgaris (the common wart). Arch Pediatr Adolesc Med. 2002 Oct;156(10):971-4.

Chapter 10: First Aid for Bumps, Bruises, and Bites

Bee Stings

Golden DB, Kagey-Sobotka A, Norman PS, Hamilton RG, Lichtenstein LM. Outcomes of allergy to insect stings in children, with and without venom immunotherapy. N Engl J Med. 2004 Aug 12;351(7):668-74.

Severino MG, Cortellini G, Bonadonna P, Francescato E, Panzini I, Macchia D, Campi P, Spadolini I, Canonica WG, Passalacqua G. Sublingual immunotherapy for large local reactions caused by honeybee sting: a double-blind, placebo-controlled trial. J Allergy Clin Immunol. 2008 Jul;122(1):44-8.

Bruises

Leu S, Havey J, White LE, Martin N, Yoo SS, Rademaker AW, Alam M. Accelerated resolution of laser-induced bruising with topical 20% arnica: a rater-blinded randomized controlled trial. Br J Dermatol. 2010 Sep;163(3):557-63.

Burns

Khorasani G, Hosseinimehr SJ, Azadbakht M, Zamani A, Mahdavi MR. Aloe versus silver sulfadiazine creams for second-degree burns: a randomized controlled study. Surg Today. 2009;39(7):587-91.

Cuts and Scrapes

Preethi KC, Kuttan R. Wound healing activity of flower extract of Calendula officinalis. J Basic Clin Physiol Pharmacol. 2009;20(1):73-9.

Dehydration

Ismail I, Singh R, Sirisinghe RG. Rehydration with sodium-enriched coconut water after exercise-induced dehydration. Southeast Asian J Trop Med Public Health. 2007 Jul;38(4):769-85.

Hives

Roschek B Jr, Fink RC, McMichael M, Alberte RS. Nettle extract (Urtica dioica) affects key receptors and enzymes associated with allergic rhinitis. Phytother Res. 2009 Jul;23(7):920-6.

Nosebleeds

Massick D, Hurtuk A. Effectiveness of a nasal saline gel in the treatment of recurrent anterior epistaxis in anticoagulated patients. Ear Nose Throat J. 2011 Sep;90(9):E4-6.

Poison Ivy

Epstein WL. Topical prevention of poison ivy/oak dermatitis. Arch Dermatol. 1989 Apr;125(4):499-501.

Wallengren J. Tea tree oil attenuates experimental contact dermatitis. Arch Dermatol Res. 2011 Jul;303(5):333-8.

Sprains

D'Anchise R, Bulitta M, Giannetti B. Comfrey extract ointment in comparison to diclofenac gel in the treatment of acute unilateral ankle sprains (distortions). Arzneimittelforschung. 2007;57(11):712-6.

Sunburn

Eberlein-König B, Placzek M, Przybilla B. Protective effect against sunburn of combined systemic ascorbic acid (vitamin C) and d-alpha-tocopherol (vitamin E). J Am Acad Dermatol. 1998 Jan;38(1):45-8.

Maenthaisong R, Chaiyakunapruk N, Niruntraporn S, Kongkaew C. The efficacy of aloe vera used for burn wound healing: a systematic review. Burns. 2007 Sep;33(6):713-8.

Chapter 11: Aches and Pains

Growing Pains

Qamar S, Akbani S, Shamim S, Khan G. Vitamin D levels in children with growing pains. J Coll Physicians Surg Pak. 2011 May;21(5):284-7.

Joint Pains

Sengupta K, Alluri KV, Satish AR, Mishra S, Golakoti T, Sarma KV, Dey D, Raychaudhuri SP. A double blind, randomized, placebo controlled study of the efficacy and safety of 5-Loxin for treatment of osteoarthritis of the knee. Arthritis Res Ther. 2008;10(4):R85.

Muscle Aches

Lyss G, Schmidt TJ, Merfort I, Pahl HL. Helenalin, an anti-inflammatory sesquiterpene lactone from Arnica, selectively inhibits transcription factor NF-kappaB. Biol Chem. 1997 Sep;378(9):951-61.

Chapter 12: Nervous System Worries

Migraine Headache

Pothmann R, Danesch U. Migraine prevention in children and adolescents: results of an open study with a special butterbur root extract. Headache. 2005 Mar;45(3):196-203.

Seizures

Tan G, Thornby J, Hammond DC, Strehl U, Canady B, Arnemann K, Kaiser DA. Meta-analysis of EEG biofeedback in treating epilepsy. Clin EEG Neurosci. 2009 Jul;40(3):173-9.

Tension Headache

Linde K, Allais G, Brinkhaus B, Manheimer E, Vickers A, White AR. Acupuncture for tension-type headache. Cochrane Database Syst Rev. 2009 Jan 21;(1):CD007587.

Tics/Tourette's Syndrome

Erickson MH. Experimental Hypnotherapy in Tourette's Disease. Am J Clin Hypn. 1965 Apr;8:325-31.

Lazarus JE, Klein SK. Nonpharmacological treatment of tics in Tourette syndrome adding videotape training to self-hypnosis. J Dev Behav Pediatr. 2010 Jul-Aug;31(6):498-504.

Chapter 13: Behavioral and Developmental Difficulties

ADHD/ADD

Fuchs T, Birbaumer N, Lutzenberger W, Gruzelier JH, Kaiser J. Neurofeedback treatment for attention-deficit/hyperactivity disorder in children: a comparison with methylphenidate. Appl Psychophysiol Biofeedback. 2003 Mar;28(1):1-12.

Gevensleben H, Holl B, Albrecht B, Vogel C, Schlamp D, Kratz O, Studer P, Rothenberger A, Moll GH, Heinrich H. Is neurofeedback an efficacious treatment for ADHD? A randomised controlled clinical trial. J Child Psychol Psychiatry. 2009 Jul;50(7):780-9.

Anger and Tantrums

Barros RM, Silver EJ, Stein RE. School recess and group classroom behavior. Pediatrics. 2009 Feb;123(2):431-6.